About the author

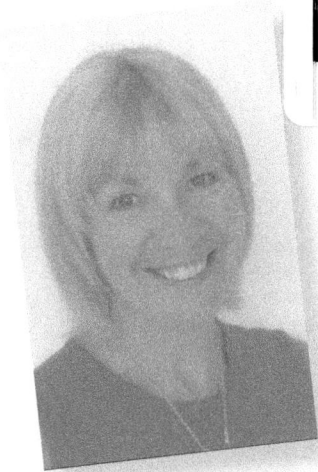

AnneMarie White is one of Australia's most respected sporting, media and entertainment personalities. Among her many accolades is a Prime Ministerial Award for 'Outstanding Media Coverage' for her contribution to women in sport. In June 2008 she was awarded the Order of Australia Medal (OAM) for her services to promoting women in sport through the media and advocacy.

During her varied career, AnneMarie has been a Media Manager at Olympic, Paralympic and Commonwealth Games and managed numerous international and national events. She was a regular on 4BC's weekly chat show, and for several years had a talk-back session on media and promotions on ABC Radio.

As an athlete, AnneMarie has represented Queensland in netball, water polo and swimming and has won several national lifesaving titles. Internationally she was ranked in the top four in Masters swimming, won a bronze medal for water polo, and competed for Australia in javelin at the 2001 World Veterans Athletics Championships.

TELLING IT LIKE IT IS

23 Breast Cancer Journeys

ANNEMARIE WHITE

ABC Books

The ABC 'Wave' device is a trademark of the
Australian Broadcasting Corporation and is used
under licence by HarperCollins*Publishers* Australia.

First published in Australia in 2009
by HarperCollins*Publishers* Australia Pty Limited
ABN 36 009 913 517
harpercollins.com.au

HarperCollins*Publishers*
25 Ryde Road, Pymble, Sydney, NSW 2073, Australia
31 View Road, Glenfield, Auckland 0627, New Zealand
A 53, Sector 57, Noida, UP, India
77–85 Fulham Palace Road, London W6 8JB, United Kingdom
2 Bloor Street East, 20th floor, Toronto, Ontario M4W 1A8, Canada
10 East 53rd Street, New York NY 10022, USA

National Library of Australia Cataloguing-in-Publication data:

White, AnneMarie
    Telling it like it is : 23 breast cancer journeys / AnneMarie White.
    ISBN 978 0 7333 2516 8 (pbk.)
    Breast – Cancer.
    Breast – Cancer – Patients – Biography.
616.99449

Cover design by Christa Moffitt, Christabella Designs
Cover illustration by iStockphoto.com
Internal design by Tango Media
Typeset in Dante MT 11.5/16pt by Letter Spaced

I dedicate this book to those amazing women and men whose journeys I have shared. I applaud their courage, their humility, their support. This book is my tribute, and this is their story.

Contents

About The National Breast Cancer Foundation

The National Breast Cancer Foundation (NBCF) is the leading community-funded national organisation in Australia supporting and promoting research into the prevention, detection and treatment of breast cancer.

Since the NBCF was established in 1994, over $55 million has been awarded to 230 research projects across every state and territory, to improve the health and wellbeing of those affected by breast cancer.

Research programs funded by the NBCF cover every aspect of breast cancer, from increasing understanding of genetics to improving ways to support women and their families.

Underpinning the NBCF's approach is the National Action Plan for Breast Cancer Research and Funding, a blueprint for accelerating our knowledge and understanding of breast cancer. The National Action Plan centres on funding collaborations with other like-minded organisations including the state based Cancer Councils and Cancer Australia. This ensures a long term, cost effective and coordinated approach to research, while providing an opportunity to accurately monitor and report outcomes to supporters.

The NBCF relies on corporate and community support to continue its work and appreciates the support of HarperCollins Publishers.

Key fundraising initiatives of the NBCF are October's Pink Ribbon campaigns, including Pink Ribbon Breakfasts, Pink Ribbon Day, Pink Magazine, Global Illumination and Pink Ribbon Licensed Product. In addition, the NBCF works with a range of corporate partners on cause-related campaigns.

The NBCF also works with third parties on major fund raising events such as the Mother's Day Classic, a national walk or run for breast cancer held annually, and reaches the youth market through the Fashion Targets Breast Cancer campaign.

Introduction

They say if you want to make God laugh, you tell her your plans ... We never really know how our lives will be lived out ... what curve balls will come out of nowhere!

In 2003, my life was as close to perfect as I could imagine — my first book, *Women Who Win*, was selling well and I was enjoying my work in media and public relations. I was fighting fit and competing with success internationally in Masters sport. I had the body and vigour of an athlete and I had signed a six-month contract to work in media in Athens at the 2004 Olympics.

On 9 May that year I was diagnosed with breast cancer. A doctor had taken me into her surgery and bluntly said, 'I guess you know you have cancer.' Timidly, I replied that I'd hoped I didn't. As it turned out I had a very aggressive Grade 3 tumour that was, fortunately, picked up early by a BreastScreen mammogram.

That weekend was Mother's Day and I gathered my family close as I looked death in the face; I'd already survived a near death experience with toxic shock, and septicaemia three years earlier in 2000. But the enormity of this horrendous disease opened the floodgates of my emotions. I was in tears, totally shocked and so scared that I was going to die. Death terrified me. Cancer is a scary word, and the reality of dying is truly frightening. It felt that my life was in tatters.

After months of chemotherapy, radiation treatment and five years of medication, I regained my health. Life was good again, and I thought I'd finished with all those curve balls. In 2007 I was celebrating my recovery from breast cancer with a zest and passion for living a great life. Then in December that year, my husband, Peter, died suddenly and unexpectedly of a massive heart attack.

With that traumatic event, the death of my soulmate of 36 years, my old wounds and fears were resurrected and came to the surface. Compounded with my grief for Peter were the memories of my own emotional moments — when I had faced my own mortality. I realised then that although I was healthy, you never really get over breast cancer. It is always there and you just live with it.

One of the ways I have chosen to make sense of where I am at, and to show gratitude for my life, is to write a book on modern-day heroes who have fought the battle against breast cancer. This book is a compendium of stories profiling the lives of a number of people who have been touched by breast cancer.

I am donating my proceeds of the book to the National Breast Cancer Foundation (NBCF) because I have no doubt that my own great health, and indeed my survival, is totally due to the advances in treatment and medication over the past years funded by the NBCF. And that is also the reason that I am honoured and proud to be an Ambassador for the NBCF.

My hope is that research breakthroughs will mean that in the future a cure for breast cancer will be found so that no one will have to travel the journey that I had to.

Hello lovely ladies

I am really looking forward to tomorrow's lunch — even more so now. But just so that this enjoyable lunch for Barbara isn't spoiled, I thought I should tell you beforehand that I have had a bit of bad news.

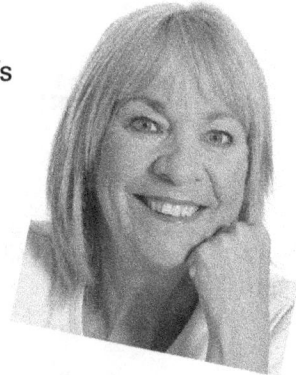

Last Friday I was diagnosed with breast cancer. Fortunately, it was done through the BreastScreen mammogram program, so it's early enough for me to be very positive. Still, facing the fact that I have a potentially fatal disease is very scary.

I am very scared and still in shock, so it will be lovely to share a meal with kind friends just before I go to my surgeon on Tuesday afternoon.

Don't worry ladies — I intend to be around, living disgracefully, well into my 90s!!!!

See you all tomorrow.

Smile (I'm still smiling!!)

AnneMarie

Taryna Michelle's Journey

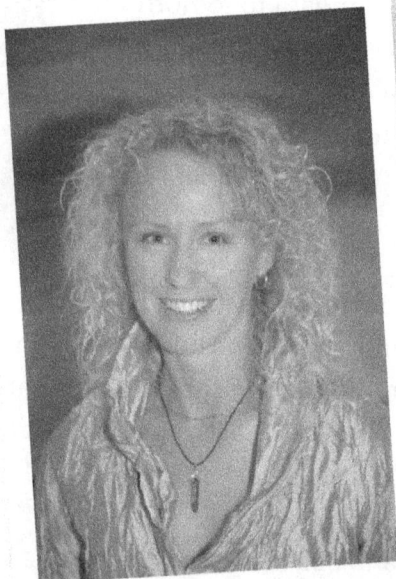

*'I had been listening to my body and I had a deep sense
that there was something wrong. So I booked in to see a
third doctor, who told me outright that there was no way it
could be anything more than an old blocked milk duct from
breastfeeding and to stop worrying.'*

From the first moment I started chatting with Taryna Michelle, a vibrant and effervescent young woman of 37, I knew she was an inspiration. She is a successful businesswoman and a mother to four girls, aged nine to 17, and life is now exciting and full of promise.

But that wasn't always so. Just four years ago Taryna felt she was living her life in a combat zone. She was diagnosed with breast cancer at only 33 and at the same time was embroiled in bitter and confrontational divorce proceedings after escaping from a volatile 13-year marriage.

Life was throwing Taryna an almighty challenge — and she was up for it.

'I didn't really know anything about breast cancer until I was diagnosed. I guess unless you are affected by it, or someone you know has it, most young people don't know too much about it. Until Kylie Minogue got cancer, there certainly wasn't much in the media; not like now. Sure, there was Melissa Etheridge and Belinda Emmett, but apart from that, as a young person, I saw breast cancer as an over-50s disease.'

Taryna's diagnosis is a story of her courage and dogged persistence when she intuitively felt that something was wrong with her body — but no one would listen.

'I've always been a big believer in listening to my body. I believe that women are very intuitive. We should always listen to our bodies and trust what it is telling us. I know now how important it is to really listen and feel!' she says emphatically.

At that time, in late 2004, she was under enormous stress in her personal life, trying to salvage what she could from the disintegration of a violent marriage to a man whom Taryna describes as difficult and belligerent. 'The constant tension was showing up in my body, and although I knew something wasn't quite right, when I look back, I realise I didn't pay enough attention to what was happening physically to me.

'I had felt a lump in my breast. That was not good, but I was also sweating profusely from one armpit and not the other. I'm

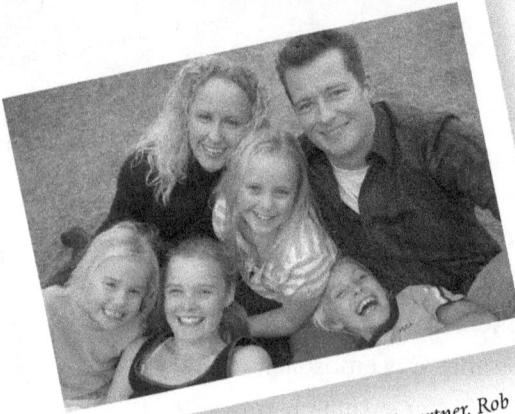
Taryna with her four daughters and partner, Rob

still not sure if the sweating thing was actually a medical indicator for breast cancer but it certainly wasn't normal for me,' Taryna says.

'In October 2004 I went to my local doctor after finding the lump and was sent off for a mammogram. The results showed that there was supposedly a bit of fatty tissue deposit but nothing to worry about. I was told I didn't need to do anything. I went home and thought, "What a relief!" But, strangely, I didn't feel relieved.'

In the following January of 2005 Taryna still had the same lump but it had grown larger. 'So I went back to the same GP, who told me I was just being a worry wart! I went home again, but as I still had the same concerns, I booked in to see a different GP.

'The next doctor also told me it was nothing and said that no one gets breast cancer at 33. Again I went home, and this time I was feeling a bit agitated. I had been listening to my body and I had a deep sense that there was something wrong. So I booked in to see a third doctor, who told me outright that there was no way it could be anything more than an old blocked milk duct from breastfeeding and to stop worrying.

'I guess I was still not happy and, because I was sure that I wasn't imagining things, I went to see yet another GP. Actually, it was my supportive partner, Rob, who pushed me to go again! This fourth doctor actually listened to me, understood my anxiety and sent me for another mammogram, a scan and a fine-needle biopsy. In fact, she was so concerned that she rang the scan place and told them to make a spot for me straight away and that it couldn't wait. She wrote out the forms and off I went, thinking, "Thank God someone finally listened!" I waited an hour in the waiting room with Rob.

'By that stage I was full of nervous anticipation! I was ushered through to the change rooms and told to take off my clothes and put on one of those very attractive robes — you know the ones … the oh-so-sexy white ones. And while we're on that subject, what the hell is the whole "three armhole" thing about? I stood there staring at it thinking two things: firstly, they must treat three-arm aliens in here pretty bloody regularly to warrant having these things and second, where are the bloody instructions for this thing?!' she laughs.

'It was 45 nerve-racking minutes, five magazines from 1982 and a very chilly tooshie later, when a lady finally comes and ushers me into an examination room, saying the radiographer will be with me soon. "Just jump up on the bed and lay down."

'Finally, I thought they would see that I was right and that they would tell me what was happening to my body.

'Another 10 minutes of waiting and in she flew — the female version of Darth Vader, parading as a radiographer. She walked straight over to me, pulled open my gown exposing my breasts and said to me, "You're wasting my time. You're 33. You don't have breast cancer. You only had a mammogram a few months ago so I am not going to do another one. I'm not doing any biopsy, either!"

'As she squirted the cold goopy stuff onto my breasts, I just lay there, dumbfounded. I felt sick. I didn't know whether to apologise or just burst out crying. I said nothing. As she roughly scanned me, I mustered up enough courage to ask her if she could see anything. She turned her head and scowled down at me. In a voice that was so angry and so cold I thought each of her words would freeze individually as they shot out of her mouth, she said, "There is nothing wrong with you. You have wasted my time. You have asymmetrical breasts." And with that, she turned sharply and left the room,' says Taryna, still dumbfounded about that offhanded treatment, even several years later.

'I just lay there, chest covered with goop, wondering if I wished hard enough, could I disappear into the cracks in the bed. The assistant to the radiographer in the room looked at me sympathetically and handed me some tissues. I cleaned myself up, got dressed and left.

'I couldn't talk to Rob at first. I was so embarrassed. I kept thinking that she was right and I had wasted everyone's time. I'd wasted Rob's time, the doctor's time, my time. I apologised to Rob and said that that was that. It was all over and there was nothing wrong.'

After Taryna's emotions had subsided, she told Rob what the radiographer had said, and he was furious. Rob wanted her to go back to the doctor but she refused.

'It took a lot of perseverance to find anyone who would take my concerns seriously, although I was nearly worn out emotionally as well as physically. But I had listened to my body and I knew something was very wrong.

'After about a week Rob basically threatened to drag me back to the doctor if I didn't go myself. The GP who had referred me called me at home then and told me to come into her surgery. I gave in and went to see her,' Taryna says.

Taryna's doctor sent her to a breast specialist who 'was completely the opposite of "Darth Radiographer". He told me that, in his experience, if a woman thought there was a problem, it was wise to listen, and testing would at the very least put the patient's mind at ease. He did say he thought that more than likely there wouldn't be any problems, but that it was always better to be safe than sorry.

'Finally, someone was empathetic! I was calm about whatever possible outcomes the tests would reveal — but I hadn't been so calm about not being able to have my concerns considered properly. When at last the breast specialist did a fine-needle biopsy and the results came back inconclusive, I knew I was right. I knew I had cancer. Even though this was serious, I felt relieved that I was on my way to having it sorted out!' Taryna recalls.

The breast specialist was very surprised. 'After the fine-needle biopsy results came back, I just remember him saying the cells were dividing and multiplying much more rapidly than normal — but at this stage he didn't know that it was cancer. He said he believed it was probably nothing, but he took the "better to be safe than sorry" line, and that's why he decided to do a lumpectomy and have a proper look.'

The results came back positive, and he looked very shocked when he broke the news to Taryna that she had DCIS — ductal carcinoma in situ.

'Telling people around me the bad news was a difficult thing to do. I was very careful of how I did that. I didn't want any negativity around me and I certainly didn't want any pity. I think I just said something like, "I don't want you to get stressed out but I've got breast cancer," and "It's going to be alright." I was really concerned about everyone around me getting anxious over it so I really played it down, like it was no big deal.

'I especially didn't want my children getting stressed out. They had already been through so much with my separation from their father and the ongoing emotional hassles associated with that. I couldn't bear to have them further upset. I think I actually felt like I had let them down by getting cancer somehow. Silly, hey?' she says, shaking her head.

'About that time I did a story on *Today Tonight* and also a double page spread in *New Idea* magazine to raise awareness about the chances of young women getting breast cancer. Rob and I were stoked to see the story in the same edition of the magazine as Bec and Lleyton Hewitt's wedding. It sold out across the country in just one week. I remember thinking that was a really great thing. Hopefully, every woman in Australia would read my story and maybe it might save lives.

'Once I was diagnosed, I just carried on as normal. I didn't have time to get upset. I was in the middle of hell with ongoing court cases with my ex-husband, who was relentless and at one stage was even threatening to have my four girls taken away from me. I knew I had to stay strong for myself and, importantly, for them. The breast cancer was just something that was going on in the background,' she says almost dismissively.

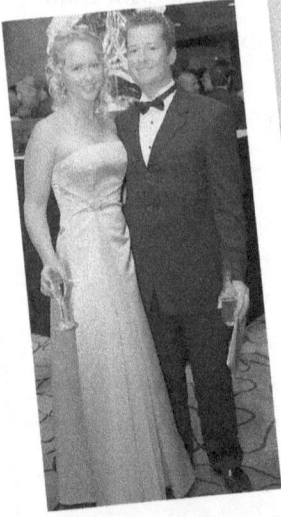

Taryna and Rob

Deciding what to do about treatments is challenging for most women, but Taryna says that her decisions were easy for her.

'I had to do everything I could to guarantee that I would be here for my kids. I wanted to have the surgery done straight away to protect my health and also because I was trying to fit in all my medical appointments around court appearances. I also saw a glimmering light somewhere in the distance that told me that I had a real chance at happiness now with Rob. I had to live! Even with all of this stuff going on, we still laughed together and planned for the future.

'Strangely, I also had this nagging feeling that there was more cancer than the doctors had found. That turned out to be right, too! It wasn't just in one place like they thought! That really proved to me the importance of listening to my body carefully,' says Taryna.

'Whilst some women may be frightened by their own mortality, I honestly never thought I was going to die. In my mind, it wasn't an option. I had stuff to do! But I have to say my greatest fear was not being there for my girls. They needed me at that time more than ever. All I knew was that I had to survive and be there for my girls.

'But I knew I wasn't going through this alone,' she says emphatically. 'My children were my inspiration. Without them, I wouldn't have soldiered on. Failure was totally out of the question. They needed me and I would never have given up on them.

'But without a shadow of a doubt, I could not have got through without Rob. He was there every single step of the way. He gave up everything he had to look after me and the girls. He lost all of his money in our business, which went down the tubes because neither of us could work in it. He lost the money he had in his house, his job, his car, everything. All to look after us. He was at every appointment with me. He stayed with me on a chair overnight every night that he could find someone to stay with the girls and then he raced home in the morning to get them up, do their hair, make their lunches and take them off to school.'

It's obvious as she speaks that Taryna has enormous gratitude for the sacrifices that Rob made. She also says that Rob's support was quite remarkable as they hadn't long been together. 'It certainly cemented our relationship, as we had only been living together for four months when I was diagnosed. The girls formed a close bond with him early on because they had to depend on him.' She asks me, 'Don't you think a family is always closer after that sort of thing?'

Once diagnosed, Taryna believes she had no other choice than to have a double mastectomy. 'I had four operations in all. Before they knocked me out for the lumpectomy I told them I had found another lump, but this time it was in the other breast. So now the doctors knew that the cancer was posing a serious threat. A double mastectomy followed the double lumpectomy. I then had reconstructions on each breast followed by what I laughingly call my jelly wobblers! All in all, seven months worth of surgeries. I reacted badly to the anaesthetic and was allergic to the painkillers, so I was in a bad way and in hospital much longer than I should have been.

'I don't think the loss of my breasts actually affected me too badly. I was looking at it as just one of those things that had to happen to ensure that I was going to be around for my girls. I also focused on the fact that I was going to get a fantastic, better-than-the-old-ones, new pair! Woo hoo! I really focused on that a lot,' she says, with a cheeky twinkle in her eyes.

Once Taryna had finished her medical journey, she concentrated on reclaiming her life and getting some sort of order back into everyday living.

'Generally speaking, I was very positive. I think I was just so relieved it was all over. I had more court stuff coming up and just kept thinking, "Now I can get this thing over and done with." I was tired for such a long time but I was never sure if it was from the breast cancer or the personal issue; it kind of blurred together. Physically, mentally and emotionally, I had love and support from Rob every step of the way. Also, because I had the girls, I needed to stay strong for them and I drew strength from them and their love for me.'

Taryna is a self-proclaimed optimist and she believes it is this sanguinity that has got her through. 'I've always been a positive person, probably overly positive sometimes, but it sure helps me move on. It's so easy to get caught up in all the small print of life, lose the bigger picture and miss out on so many opportunities — you know, the whole "Can't see the forest for the trees" thing. I love that saying!' she says brightly.

'At the risk of sounding a little cheesy, I always find time to laugh and never, ever have any regrets. I look for the humour in a situation and if I can't find any, then I ask myself what I learned from it. I always get into so much trouble from my girls when I say this. Actually, it drives them nuts! But I just think of that lesson as the taxi that's going to take me from where I am now to where I want to be. Post-breast cancer, I am definitely more confident. I think that no matter how big or small most events are in your life, each one changes you; it's only the degree that differs.'

Then, after a thoughtful pause, she adds candidly, 'I honestly think that all the bad stuff I went through with my ex gave me the strength to get through the cancer. I remember thinking to myself that it took me so long to get the courage to finally leave the marriage, and that if I could do that, I could survive breast cancer, no worries — piece of cake! I'm really looking forward to the next part of my life now, with Rob and the girls. Good times ahead!'

Taryna's incredibly cheerful outlook on life didn't just magically appear. It was a state of mind that she worked very hard to achieve as she knew it would be mental toughness that would carry her through.

'I'm a lot more self-confident these days. I had to tell myself so often that I was a strong, confident woman who could survive this and anything else that was thrown at me that I guess I ended up believing it.'

Today, after having survived so much — the many emotional upheavals of her breast cancer journey at a young age; a bitter divorce battle; two business failures, because she didn't have enough working time — Taryna says she is a changed person with a bright future beckoning.

'Rob and I launched Funktown — a print business — and then CrazyBird — a graphic design business. We created them with the philosophy that we would only work with people who were truly kind and would refuse to do business with people who were rude, mean, aggressive or anything other than just plain nice! We are working really hard and I admit it is a struggle to keep it going. But again, it's that positive attitude that will make it work,' she states confidently.

Taryna is also dedicated to promoting breast cancer awareness in young women, speaking at a wide variety of functions and events in Western Australia. 'I've got one coming up in a pole-dancing fitness studio next week! That should be heaps of fun. I can do the message — don't know about the pole,' she laughs.

She says, 'I'm not a professional speaker. I'm not trained. I'm just a mum, a partner, a sister, a friend, trying to get an important message across. I tell those in the audiences to listen to their own body and if they have persistent niggles or concerns, then follow them through. After my own experience of trying to get someone to take me seriously at 33, I also tell people to never give up.

'Photography has always been a hobby of mine, but I've never had the nerve to do anything about it — until now. I have a camera that I really love using and I am starting to take more photos. I even shot a wedding recently and had such a ball. I hope I can continue taking photographs professionally. I would also really like to take the creative side of my photography further and put together a book of photos of survivors from all over Australia, all different ages and backgrounds — happy photos for people to draw strength from. Rob has even created a website to showcase my photos,' she adds.

With what she hopes was the last of the four-year-long legal proceedings through the family court concluded four months ago, Taryna is now ready to start her own personal healing process.

'When I was going through my breast cancer treatments I was too busy looking after everyone else and I guess I neglected myself. But now I have put my past behind me and I am focusing on me a little more,' she says confidently.

'Finally, the time has come to heal myself. I have joined a gym and three days a week I work out for an hour. I recognise I can only repair my physical body and restore my mental and emotional health with a little more *me* time.

'With that recovery comes a new energy, a zest for life and an optimism that I hope will nurse me back to good health and ensure a new and prosperous future,' she says.

After a minefield of trouble and a bucketload of challenges, life is good once again for this young woman.

Lovely ladies,

Thanks for your prayers and guardian angels. They worked.
I'm alive!

Finally got out of the hospital, although I still have a couple
of full body scans on Wednesday. Thought I'd respond to you
lovely people who took the time to care for me with your
prayers, best wishes and phone calls.

The good news is the surgeon did a great job of cutting out
all the cancer and the margins were well clear. The best news
was that there was no movement through the lymph system
and only 4 nodes were taken out.

The scary news is that it was graded as a virulent 3. That is
the strongest and most aggressive form of breast cancer ...
usually reserved for much younger people. I always knew
that I was younger than my chronological age but gee, didn't
need proof this way!

The absolutely blessed thing, though, is that because I
was speaking up north in Port Douglas, I had delayed my
bi-annual mammogram by 10 weeks. The surgeon can't be
sure but he feels that because the cancer was very tiny — but
grew so quickly — had I had the mammogram at the earlier
time, it just may not have been detected and I could have
been dead before it was found! So God obviously wants me
here for some reason.

The outcome is that I start chemo on June 6th and such is the strength of the chemo cocktail that I'll probably lose my hair within days. Just as well I wear it short, hey? After 6 months of that I do 2 months of radiotherapy and then drugs for the next few years.

I'm speaking at the Queensland Businesswomen's Breakfast on the 5th at the Royal on the Park. So if you are free that morning, it would be beautiful to see some friendly faces in the audience.

At the moment it seems I'll never get my life back — or that I will have an obsession about medical matters forever. But being an optimist, I figure the bouts of crying and feelings of overwhelming helplessness will soon be replaced by my irrepressible spirit. I still want to be a disgraceful old lady at 94!!

The oncologist reckons I am the best news story for breast screening they have at the moment!!! Geoff Heugill is doing a 'shave off' with the cancer kids at the hospital for me in a week or so. Maybe we can do the oncology shave together?

Thanks again for your love. Knowing that I have friends who will be there for me over the coming year gives me strength and courage.

Smile — I still am!

AM

Fiona Stanley's Journey

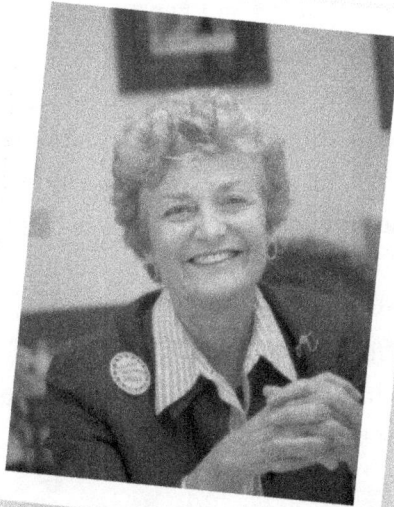

'I went through all of the questions: "Why me?"
"Why did this happen to me?" "What did I do wrong?"
"Was there something I could have done?"'

$\mathcal{P}$rofessor Fiona Stanley AC is passionate about the health of Australians — in particular, the children. She is the founding Director of the Telethon Institute for Child Health Research in Western Australia, Executive Director of the Australian Research Alliance for Children and Youth, and Professor in the School of Paediatrics and Child Health at the University of Western Australia.

She has dedicated her life to researching the causes of major childhood illnesses and birth defects. In 1996 she was awarded a Companion of the Order of Australia and then in 2003, in recognition of her outstanding dedication and contributions to the nation, she was named Australian of the Year.

Fiona strongly believes that we must 'get things right' for children and families now, so we can look towards a positive and healthy future for Australia. But back in 1999 it was Fiona who had to look to her own positive and healthy future when she was diagnosed with breast cancer.

She remembers being extremely angry. 'I just didn't want this; I didn't have time for this. Actually it was quite strange because I didn't worry about having cancer as much as feel annoyed about this imposition that was thrust upon me when I had so much else to do in my life,' she says.

She found the lump when she took some time off to move house. At the time, she says, 'I wasn't feeling particularly brilliant about lots of things and decided to go and have a check-up with my GP.' She admits that it's not often that doctors go to doctors, and they don't go and have regular check-ups. 'But I was extremely grateful that I had listened to that inner voice telling me to go for the check-up. When I went to my GP, she found the lump and then she told me not to delay in getting it ultrasounded. "Do it straight away," she urged.'

It had been 11 months since Fiona's last mammogram and she didn't think that the lump was going to be anything sinister. She rationalised, 'Oh well, 90 per cent of lumps are not malignant, so I'm going to be okay. But I went pretty quickly — not really from a sense of nervous urgency but because I just wanted to get this out of the way. Really, it was because I just needed to know.

'I wasn't particularly worried at that stage. But as soon as I hit the ultrasound place and they sort of raced me into an emergency mammogram and then started talking about which oncologist I needed to choose, I realised that it was very serious — especially as the person doing the ultrasound and the woman doing the emergency mammogram were both pretty confident that this was a malignant lesion,' says Fiona.

Being an epidemiologist, Fiona knew her way around medical testing and procedures, but was still disappointed with the information she was given, and wonders about how women without her background and experience deal with the diagnostic process.

'It's interesting, actually, and I've thought about this quite a lot. If I found some of this difficult, how does Ms Average find it? I guess that was going through my mind. Not only do I keep up a little bit with the literature on breast cancer — because it's just something that one does in the reading of journals — but also, being a doctor, they obviously treated me differently. And I know that I wanted more information. I still feel dissatisfied with the information given to me at that time,' she says.

Ironically, Fiona had been on the Health Care Committee for the National Health and Medical Research Council that produced what she describes as a superb series of booklets on breast cancer. 'I read them that first night and they really helped me understand my situation.'

However, whilst she is a little critical of the level of information she was given, Fiona is enthusiastic in her appreciation of the speed with which her tumour analysis was returned to her.

'That part of my diagnosis was reassuring. I had a needle biopsy straight away in the morning and by that night I knew not only that I had a malignant tumour, but that it was a middle-of-the-road kind of aggressive cancer. I thought that was superb in terms of the rapidity of diagnosis and not having to wait too long. That was unlike the experience of my sister-in-law, who happens to live in New York, the great American environment. She had a breast lump at the same time and had, I think, a very inferior diagnostic work-up to me. She had to wait two weeks before she had a biopsy. Fortunately, her lump was not malignant.'

Once Fiona had the biopsy she returned to the office to wait for the phone call. 'I tried to not think about it and just threw myself into my work. But I must confess I was feeling incredibly worried; I was terribly, terribly anxious.

'Strangely, apart from my husband, Geoff, who was understandably also very worried, I didn't know who to tell because at an emotionally challenging time like this there are so many things going on around you. But at the same time I was also very aware that just because I was getting breast cancer, it doesn't mean that things stopped happening. One of my daughters was sitting for her final exams for university entrance and my other daughter was doing her final university exams. I didn't know whether to tell them or not. So I didn't for nearly a week.

'I don't actually know how my daughters really felt about my cancer — looking back now at that time, I think they were really scared inside but keen to give me all the positive support that they could.'

After she received the diagnosis on Tuesday afternoon, she had to decide who would perform the surgery. As she is part of the medical fraternity, Fiona knew who was who in Western Australia. 'I knew there were many very good surgeons here, so I chose somebody who I knew was also very nice and would be a good person to talk to. I've also had such a good result from surgery because I chose a surgeon who took breast cancer as one of his specialties,' she says.

She delayed having surgery till the following Monday 'because we were actually moving house on the Friday. Moving house paled into insignificance compared with this. But it was a distraction and so, in some sense, it was quite a good way of moving house.'

The family was, as expected, in total shock. 'And I think that was the sort of response from everybody I talked to. By this time I was actually getting accustomed to the fact that I had breast cancer, and so I tended to find myself comforting people about it and saying, "Well, it's really okay."'

I've talked with a large cross-section of women diagnosed with breast cancer and it seems that women deal with diagnosis by becoming the strong one — and Fiona was no exception. 'You sort of go round comforting people about your own disease. It's sort of strange, but that's exactly what happened to me. I would keep telling people not to worry because this cancer isn't going to beat me. I stayed strong but everyone I spoke to burst into tears.'

However, it wasn't long before Fiona's own tears flowed. She was in hospital preparing for the operation. 'Stupidly, I hadn't arranged to have anyone wait with me on the morning before the surgery. I was alone and got terribly anxious before I had the pre-med. But just when I thought I couldn't cope, my eldest daughter walked in and held my hand, and we sat there talking. She was fantastic, and it certainly helped me get through that terrible period of waiting.'

Her hospital stay also proved to be an emotional time. 'Every morning I woke very early, terribly upset and in tears. I had to ring my friends in the eastern States because I couldn't get anyone at home — it was four o'clock in the morning here. So there I was on the phone ringing my friends in Melbourne for company, reassurance and comfort.'

Friends proved to be an enormous encouragement for Fiona, and she is clearly still appreciative of all the help and love she received. 'I had a most extraordinary amount of support from my friends. I remember the flowers in the hospital went all the way around my room and down the corridor! One of my work colleagues cooked a gourmet meal every Saturday for the whole six months I was on chemotherapy. There was a roster at work to support and cook for us. My friends were wonderful and loving. My Aboriginal friends were so supportive and gave me traditional healing remedies and collected special bush medicine to strengthen me — I was literally overwhelmed.'

'I felt that I had to get better because so many people were so wonderful and I couldn't let them down! In 1999 breast cancer was not quite as common as it is now and it seems to me that the outcomes were more scary — now it appears more commonplace, and the results are so good for many. Perhaps if it had happened now, people would not be as concerned.'

Fiona also owns up to still being angry at that time. 'There was a resentment that remained there: a sense of unfairness that I had got cancer and about all of those associated challenges that were happening to me,' she says. 'Getting over this anger took some time. Even 12 months later I still felt quite depressed and actually sought some counselling, which helped. I also did a creative writing day, which was like a healing workshop. Gradually I was able to move on and found it progressively easier to resume my own life.

'That has now passed and I'm pretty much adapted to the fact that breast cancer was something that I had to have and I'm going to be okay.'

Added to this disquiet, Fiona faced the 'what ifs' — those questions with the potent combination of fear, apprehension and anger which can rarely be answered, yet plague women at this time of their lowest physical and emotional resistance. 'I went through all of the questions: "Why me?" "Why did this happen to me?" "What did I do wrong?" "Was there something I could have done?"' she admits.

Fiona was particularly curious and fretful about the fact she had been taking HRT prior to her diagnosis. 'Did I get breast cancer because I'd been on hormone replacement therapy? As a woman, that concern kept coming back to haunt me, and I know other women must feel the same. As an epidemiologist in causal pathways, I am extremely interested and indeed need to have answers.'

Fiona says she is almost totally convinced that HRT influenced the rate of growth of her cancer but remains undecided about whether it was the trigger. 'Studies have come out recently which support that explanation. I would advise women now to only go on a short course of HRT or not to have it at all,' she adds.

Fiona had a successful quadrantectomy and an axillary clearance surgery, which meant that because the lump was quite large, the surgeon cut out a section of the breast rather than just the lump itself. She had no lymph node involvement — for which she is grateful, saying, 'They were all negative. You see, I'm in a very low-risk group, so in so many ways I'm very lucky.'

Fiona's next challenge was chemotherapy, a step she only decided upon after careful consideration. 'It was because I believed that chemotherapy really did reduce the risk of recurrence quite dramatically. But I concede that there was also a combination of fear and anger. Not particularly a fear of death — that didn't worry me; it was fear of actually being ill, being ill on chemo.

'The good thing about breast cancer is the research that's been done at the moment. And, of course, being an epidemiologist, I got straight into researching what was being written about chemotherapy. Just by chance, the week that I was deciding whether to have chemotherapy, the biggest systematic review of the literature analysis was published in the UK, in the *British Medical Journal*.

'From my reading, I could see that there had been a huge set of trials, and it looked like everybody benefited from chemotherapy, so there really wasn't any debate for me. Even knowing all that, going into my first chemotherapy session I was absolutely petrified. I think I'm a wimp, basically, and I was scared,' she owns up.

Fiona is also the first to acknowledge that she was really lucky. 'My reaction to chemotherapy was mostly just feeling a bit nauseated and very fatigued. It kind of flattened me. I couldn't do anything much, which is very unacceptable to me. I hate not being able to do things, so I'm not very good at just lying around.'

Whilst other women lose their hair and have many more gut complications than Fiona did during her treatment, she did have several unusual reactions: 'Funny things, like I got severe infections under my fingernails and I had difficulty with vision; I couldn't read properly all the time.

'But compared to others, I was extremely lucky during my chemo treatments,' she says. 'I had a major adverse reaction to the anti-nausea tablets, which was ghastly, but improved after changing to a new drug. The Cancer Foundation ran these marvellous classes in meditation, nutrition, make-up and hair care etc — I went to all of them and really found them fantastic.'

Radiotherapy was not a pleasant experience for Fiona, who suffered from radiation burns and fatigue. 'I disliked the radiotherapy because you are alone in a room with a machine which is still like equipment that was used in the 1940s for cancer treatments. It made me feel quite scared and vulnerable,' she admits.

Reflecting back on her months of treatment, Fiona is clear that the one thing that could have been improved for her was the coordination of care. She explains: 'Individually, each of the therapists — the surgeon, the oncologist in charge of the chemotherapy and the radiation oncologist — was terrific, as were the nurses. In fact, the nurses were absolutely superb in the way they delivered the chemo and helped with my radiation burns. And they really cared very deeply about my comfort. But it's just that if you get a complication — and I had some quite nasty side effects and complications with some of the therapies — you don't know who to go to.

'There was no one person sitting across your care who, if you saw him or her once a week, would ask, "How are you going? What do you need now?" I did feel I was on my own.

'I remember the old-fashioned case conferences that we used to have when I was doing clinical medicine. When you were dealing with a multi-system or multi-specialty disease, everyone came together and said, "Well, this is the plan for this person." And I think the concept of having someone assess you and then decide on who you need to see or what you need to do is a good one. The concept of having a breast cancer nurse coordinator to do that would be a great idea,' she suggests.

Others may feel that a woman's GP can fulfil that role. With the benefit of hindsight, Fiona concedes that she could have made her somewhat horrendous breast cancer journey easier for herself had she worked more closely with her GP. 'I think the GP who found my lump is my heroine. I mean, she's fantastic. And to a certain extent I excluded her, I guess, because I was racing around thinking, "I've got to find the best person and it's got to be done now." In fact, I should have sat down with her and spent some more time working things out.'

Ten years on from her diagnosis, Fiona says that she looks after her health more these days 'but not just because of the breast cancer. It is because I am now 62 and I want to be as healthy as possible in my older years. I exercise regularly, do yoga, juice often and try and have really good holidays.'

Fiona is now very engaged with her work and doesn't dwell on her breast cancer experience. 'It seems odd that others think that I have had a life-threatening experience, and yes, maybe I have, but I just don't look on it like that. I realise that life is eventually fatal and we all have to come to terms with that — I don't really think about it much now,' she says.

'It is strange that my work life, if anything, has become more demanding not less since I had breast cancer. I haven't done this intentionally. It is just that a lot of important things needed to happen at work both in Perth and nationally.'

And with the construction under way in Perth of the new 643-bed Fiona Stanley Hospital, named after this eminent Western Australian doctor and Australian of the Year, Fiona moves on from her trials with breast cancer to a multitude of new challenges, including ensuring health protection for Aboriginal children and continuing her role as UNICEF Australia Ambassador for Early Childhood Development.

From: AnneMarie
Subject: FOAMs
Sent: 5 June 2003

Beautiful FOAMs

The FOAMs are born! (FOAMs stand for **Friends of AnneMarie!**)

Let me give you all a huge electronic hug for supporting me at the Businesswomen's Breakfast this morning. As you know, I had accepted the speaking engagement months ago — long before I was diagnosed with breast cancer.

Stepping up in front of an audience of 400 is always daunting. But in the fragile emotional state I'm in at the moment, this was always going to be a very tough challenge.

You will never really know how much your individual attendance meant to me and how the 'standing ovation' totally humbled me. Thank you so much, dear FOAMs.

Late today what I had known informally for a day or so was confirmed — that my chemo has been delayed a week and is now rescheduled for Friday 13th, Black Friday — so any errant cancer cells beware!

This was a huge emotional blow as I has prepared myself physically and mentally for tomorrow. However *in God's time not mine* seems appropriate in this instance. I remember how timing saved my life earlier in this mini saga. I look on the next week as a gift to relax and to prepare again.

And hey, I have another week of hair and drinking!!!

Smile ... I am!

Love you all.

AM

Kerryn McCann's Journey

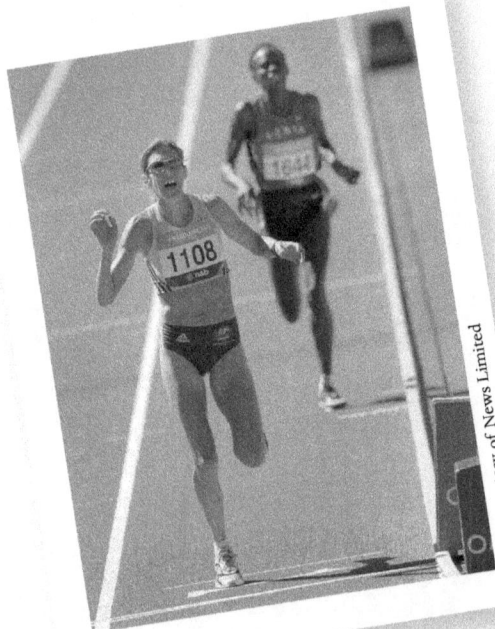

'I did do stories for papers, and television for National Breast Cancer Awareness week. I wanted to help people be aware that it could happen to them and to tell women to get in early for scans if a lump is found, so that it can be detected early for better results.'

She was the hero of the 2006 Commonwealth Games in Melbourne. Her fierce confrontation with Kenya's Hellen Cherono in the final stages of the women's marathon will go down in Australian sporting history as one of the epic battles in athletics. But it is Kerryn McCann's battle with deadly breast cancer that cemented her status as an Australian legend.

I watched that March day in 2006 from the sidelines, with hundreds of other screaming fans, as the gritty Australian athlete ran down the railroad ramp ahead of Cherono. Turning into the Melbourne Cricket Ground, she was overtaken by her dogged rival as we spectators roared encouragement. The lead changed many times before Kerryn McCann crossed the finish line two seconds ahead of Cherono to remain the Commonwealth Queen of the Marathon — a title she had earned four years earlier in Manchester.

At the time, a relieved and triumphant Kerryn told Australia, 'That wasn't me running that last 300 metres. I think it's probably the greatest victory I've ever had, or the greatest race I've ever run.'

Eighteen months later, she was again lining up for a marathon — but of another kind, telling Australia, 'I have breast cancer.'

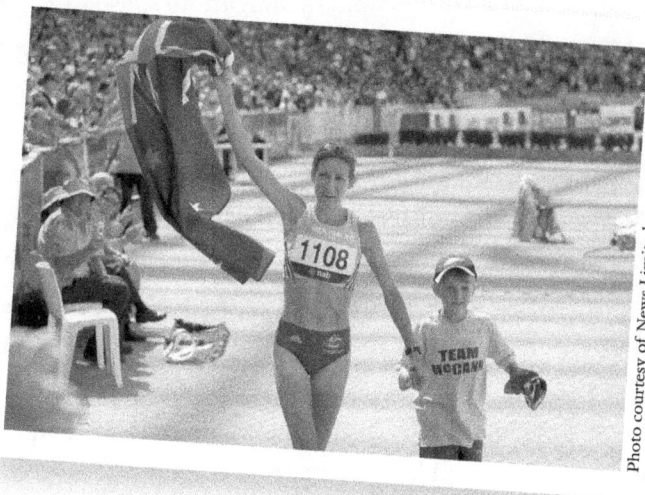

Kerryn with son Benton after winning in 2006

When I visit Kerryn McCann to interview her for this book, her fighting spirit is strongly evident. No challenge is too great to face; no race too hard to run. And her battle against breast cancer is one she is determined to win. 'I am ready to fight it,' she tells me.

Breast cancer was not really something Kerryn knew much about before her own diagnosis. 'I went to a fair few fundraisers for women suffering with breast cancer and I really felt for those women. Little did I know that would be me later on.

'When I was asked in interviews to describe my life before my diagnosis, I could sum it up in one word: perfect. I have often said my life was so good it scared me. I loved what I have and was — and indeed still am — thankful for my beautiful family and friends. Life for us was fun, full of adventures, lots of holidays. I guess, like a lot of people, it was busy but fun.'

In 2007 Kerryn was pregnant with her third child when she went to her doctor with what she had dismissed as a minor lump in her breast. 'I thought I had a blocked milk duct and when it kept growing, I was worried it may affect me breastfeeding my baby. That was the reason why I mentioned it to my doctor — so I could get the blocked duct fixed before the baby came along. I had no idea there was anything wrong with me or anything more sinister than a minor blocked duct,' Kerryn explains.

However, the harsh reality of breast cancer was looming.

'At my first ultrasound, the nurse was very chatty and said she would send the results off and the doctor would get them sometime next week. Then, while ultrasounding the lump, she called the doctor in, who asked a lot of questions about the lump, then asked if breast cancer was in my family. They told me the results would be faxed that afternoon and ready to be picked up in an hour. "A benign or malignant tumour" was what was written on the report.

'I was angry after I left because I thought they were making me worry over nothing, and here I was pregnant. I didn't need the extra worry,' she says.

Even though she sees herself as a pragmatic person, Kerryn was agitated enough to have a sleepless night. 'But,' she says, 'I believed I was probably overreacting and everything would be okay.' But all was not okay.

'I had a biopsy. The next day I was told by my gynaecologist at the hospital that the lump was a malignant tumour and that it needed to be treated immediately.

'I was booked in the following day to see an oncologist, and he, too, was in a panic. He agreed that the tumour needed treating right away but he wanted to give me chemotherapy first to shrink the lump. The news was all bad. He told me that the growth was stuck on the chest wall and that it would be hard to remove it all.

'He continued to tell me that it was an aggressive Grade 3 cancer, and that I would have to go through chemotherapy. The only good news was that the cancer cells were detected in only one lymph node. I was shocked, but my husband, Greg, started to sweat and had to lean on the table. He almost fainted. He picked up the phone and started calling the doctors in front of us,' Kerryn says.

As Kerryn was pregnant, decisions about treatment — tough enough for anyone dealing with a cancer diagnosis — became even harder for her and Greg to make. Ensuring the protection of her unborn child was uppermost in Kerryn's mind, but she and her husband were also faced with the urgency of arresting the growth of her aggressive cancer. The steely athlete was facing a tumultuous rollercoaster of emotions.

'I said to my oncologist I didn't care what he did as long as I lived. Together we would do what was best for me and my baby.

'At this time I was 31 weeks pregnant, and my gynaecologist had said no to chemo, fearing it may harm my unborn baby. The good news was that my surgeon said he could feel the lump and he was confident he could get it all out. We went with the surgeon's decision and I had the lump cut out the next day.

'I prayed the surgeon would get it all and I tried to be positive. I woke up after surgery and anxiously asked the surgeon if he had got it all. Thankfully he said yes he had and so I ticked off the first hurdle,' a relieved Kerryn says. 'Once I found out the surgeon had got it all and the oncologist said the chemo was now a mop-up job, I finally could sleep.

'After surgery I was a little sore but I recovered quickly. At first I was upset that I'd lost part of my breast but I sort of got used to it. After all, it is a small price to pay for your life, isn't it?' she asks.

So that Kerryn could have treatment as soon as possible, Kerryn and Greg's little baby boy, Cooper, was induced six weeks early and was delivered naturally on Wednesday 5 September 2007 at 11.15pm.

Kerryn had scans done the next morning at 10am — only 11 hours after giving birth — and again the following day. As they were clear, chemotherapy was scheduled to start on the following Monday.

'It was very hard because Cooper was six weeks premature so he had to stay in hospital for three weeks. We travelled into the hospital every morning and every night to see him. I hated seeing him hooked up to all the tubes and drips; I felt guilty that he was brought into the world too soon and that I wasn't even allowed to breastfeed him — not even for that special first night — because of the scans I had to have the next day,' explains an emotional Kerryn.

'It was a difficult few weeks until he came home to the family. Then it felt better and normal for us to be looking after him in our own home, rather than the nurses in hospital. Although I have to say that the nurses were fantastic.'

Kerryn reveals that at first she was scared of the medical fraternity 'because they had so much bad news. I didn't know what I should do or what treatments I should be having. I couldn't make any of those dreadfully hard decisions; I had no idea. So I let the doctors make them for me — doing what was best for me. And I did what I was told,' she says.

'Once the good results came back after surgery, my outlook changed to be much more positive. I think the medical staff are all fantastic and really know so much about breast cancer. I trusted them and believe in them. The oncologist said he knew the type of cancer

I was diagnosed with and had had success with it. It wasn't a popular cancer but he got me through,' she adds.

Kerryn was scheduled to have six chemotherapy treatments spaced three weeks apart followed by six weeks of radiotherapy. Resolute, she just got on with the treatment. 'I really didn't have any reservations about having chemo as this was what the doctors advised. So once the decision was made for me to have chemo, I couldn't wait for it to start. I just wanted to get on with it and get it over with.

'At first I hated all those harsh chemicals going through my healthy body and couldn't help but think how bad this poison was. But I grew to believe that it does its job in killing off all the bad cells. I took the philosophy that I would be healthy again once it was finished. While in training, I wouldn't even take an anti-inflammatory pill because of what it may do to my insides so when they gave me steroids to stop the sickness I was horrified.

'My first chemo session was five days after giving birth to Cooper. I got back pains so was given a relaxant, and it helped immediately. It took four hours for the first chemo treatment to be injected into my veins. I ached that night and I couldn't sleep, but I would say that was because I had just given birth. The next two treatments were a breeze but number 4 knocked me flat. I felt like I had morning sickness all over again plus a virus. I was very tired and weak and struggled to pick up my baby, so my husband did everything for those few days after the treatment. I would then recover and feel fine up until the next one,' Kerryn says.

'The worst bit about chemo was the days immediately after each treatment. This was the only time I took medication — which I didn't like taking. I seemed to be tired and sick but then I'd get better. I guess I can't complain. The worst is the tiredness. My husband had to do everything, which was hard for me because I feel like it is my job. It is hard letting people do things for me when I'm used to doing everything. But I was also very grateful for all the support and help I did get. My friends and family made a roster to cook for me every week. Another good friend cleans as well. I am so lucky to have true friends,' says Kerryn.

Although completely grateful that she is alive, well and powering back to an active and positive life, she says, 'During chemotherapy, when I wasn't feeling well, I sometimes felt a bit helpless and depressed. I got better, though, as the weeks passed. Before I was diagnosed I was running, but afterwards I wasn't allowed to run because of the iron/haemoglobin deficiency. That was hard, too — not feeling fit and healthy.

'I had read a lot of information on what to expect so I really thought I would feel worse. But I think my fitness helped with my recovery. I do admit to worrying that chemo might not work but I am thankful now for every single day.'

Following chemotherapy Kerryn faced two months of radiation treatments. 'Radiotherapy was a breeze compared to the chemo. They said I would feel very tired but I didn't feel tired at all. My only complaint was my terribly burned skin. It was very sore and bright red and the skin blistered. I was told this would happen so it was no great surprise,' she says.

Looking back now at those first days of diagnosis, Kerryn remembers she not only had to deal with her own personal anguish but, as she was such a popular athletic champion, she was forced into sharing her journey with the public. 'I told my mum first that I was having scans. Then I rang my dad, who was hysterical. I felt guilty I hadn't mentioned that there could be something wrong, but I didn't want to make a big deal of it in case it turned out to be nothing. My sister was next and Greg's mum. They probably had a fair idea, though, that something serious was wrong because of the rush through the week with medical appointments, ultrasounds and biopsies,' she recalls.

'Once I knew I had breast cancer I rang close family. But I found it too hard to tell my friends so I texted them, I wrote: "Don't ring me, too upset to speak right now, I'll ring you, I have breast cancer."

'I tried to keep it from the public but I had commitments

throughout the rest of the year with sponsors like Anlene and event organisers like the Melbourne Marathon. Word got out. I was really upset that the media were so upfront and inquisitive,' Kerryn adds.

'But in spite of that, I did do stories for papers, and television for National Breast Cancer Awareness week. I wanted to help people be aware that it could happen to them and to tell women to get in early for scans if a lump is found, so that it can be detected early for better results,' says Kerryn. 'I felt that I could use my profile to perhaps help other women.

'I have had a lot of contact with people such as Jane McGrath and Raelene Boyle who have been diagnosed with breast cancer and who also have gone through the same public scrutiny. I found it a great help to me, speaking with such strong and inspirational women. They have helped me to be strong.

'They were terribly supportive and gave me great advice. I remember Jane telling me to stop going on the internet all the time. She made me promise I would stop that — and I did. It is true. You read too many bad things and they seem to stick with you. So I now tell others to read only good positive things because they help you be positive and that helps in your recovery.

'I love hearing good stories about people who were worse off than me but have overcome adversity and live a normal healthy life again. I read Lance Armstrong's books. His is such a positive story,' says Kerryn.

'But being strong didn't mean that I didn't still worry — my greatest fear was leaving my family behind: my kids, my unborn baby, my husband. During this whole ordeal, they have all been there for me every single step of the way,' Kerryn says, with emotion creeping into her voice. 'Like me, everyone close to me was shocked and upset, but then they became my rock — strong and confident, supportive.

'My husband's strength — his love and support and his reassurance — keep me going. He has taken time off work to look after me, the kids and baby Cooper. I would be stuck without him.

My mum is also great. She's always there and helps me cope with all my fears and tears.'

For every person diagnosed with cancer, thoughts of facing death open the emotional floodgates. Kerryn was no different. 'At first you are in shock and then you become more practical. I made plans, I gathered my family close. We prayed, we bargained with God, and then we just had to wait.

'I guess I had a fair idea in the beginning that the breast cancer was potentially fatal, but I was more upset when I didn't know where I stood. Once I found out and could do something about it, I coped a little better. It was the hardest three weeks of my life and yes, I did a lot of praying. I thought the worst — only natural, isn't it? I cried a hell of a lot,' Kerryn confesses.

But out of the intense turbulence of emotions, fears and panic attacks, there always appear some gifts. 'Amidst all the bad news my husband and I learned how strong our love for each other is. This shock also makes me appreciate everything I have and do. Now I try not to be worrying about petty things,' Kerryn says philosophically.

'The other wonderful gift from my diagnosis has been the terrific support of my friends. They can't do enough for me now. Sometimes I find that hard to accept. But as my sister told me, "You would do the same for them." And she is right. I love my friends and would help them if they needed it. They keep telling me that they help me for their own sake because that is all they can do. It helps them feel better knowing that they are doing something for me.

'And they have all now gone out and had mammograms. They were all in shock that someone like myself — fit and healthy — could get breast cancer. So that's another positive.'

And of course, from time to time the seriousness of this medical war against breast cancer is lightened with humorous moments.

'I remember watching my son in the pool from my balcony, and the wind blew off my wig. I scrambled around the balcony grabbing at my wig before it blew away — and especially before the neighbours saw my bald head. I finally got it back and put it on my head and looked down to see my 10-year-old son rolling around on the ground in hysterical laughter. So of course I just went into fits of laughter, too. We have the same sense of humour; we laugh at others' misfortunes.'

Now that she has been through her treatments and is able to reflect on her experiences, Kerryn does admit to some frustration and irritation about the intrusion of cancer into her life. However, putting that behind her, she is now totally refocused on living a healthy life.

'I have to see my oncologist every three months and have scans every year. But I am not worried about it coming back because I've been told there is a 97 per cent survival rate for breast cancer. I believe in being positive. It's silly to worry about something that will probably never happen,' Kerryn says.

'Although it is not so long since my journey with breast cancer, I think I am coping quite well — physically, mentally and emotionally. I have learned so much from two inspirational women: Jane McGrath and Raelene Boyle. They have helped me to not be scared any more.

'I don't have time to worry: having three children, and one being only six months old, I'm too busy to think about it. People have said how bad the timing was — being pregnant and having breast cancer — but I think it was a blessing. Whenever I was feeling really sick, I would lie down with Cooper while he slept and just stare at his beautiful little face, and it made me feel so good. He is a beautiful boy and I feel so lucky,' she says.

Kerryn's secret to getting on with her life is simple. 'I'm back running and feeling fit and healthy again. I feel strong when I run. It's normal to me and I want everything to be back to normal. I have goals and I think that helps in my recovery. My goals aren't as high as they were, but it's nice to set smaller goals and work towards achieving them. I like to keep busy; it gives me something to think about. I just want to have fun now, with my family and friends.'

Kerryn McCann was an admired figure in Australia even before she was struck down with breast cancer. Since her diagnosis and subsequent treatments, she has earned the respect of the nation: not only is she a champion runner, she's a true inspiration. If life is like a marathon race, then Kerryn is again showing her championship form.

Perhaps it will be her battle against breast cancer that is 'the greatest victory I have had and the greatest race I have ever run'.

POSTSCRIPT: 8 DECEMBER 2008

Kez is in Heaven

With that simple text message, Greg McCann let family and friends know that his beloved wife, Kerryn, had run the last lap of her life and had crossed the finishing line.

In September 2008 Kerryn had stated that she was undergoing 'a few problems', as she was stricken with secondary cancer in her liver. She died at age 41, surrounded by Greg and their children: Benton, 11, Josie, 5, and baby Cooper, just 14 months old.

Kerryn will be remembered for being a champion athlete but for much more besides. Her dignity and courage in winning races and in fighting breast cancer has touched all Australians.

We will remember the woman who fought with everything she had — until her final breath.

From: AnneMarie
Subject: DISAPPOINTING NEWS TODAY
Sent: 10 June 2003

Hello everyone

Just thought I'd share my frustrations with you tonight. I'd
delayed starting my chemo because I thought I was going
to be able to take part in an international breast cancer drug
trial. Now, after waiting for 3 weeks while my paperwork was
processed in America and France, I was told this morning I
am not eligible for the trial after all!

And this is all for the sake of 2 nodules! My surgeon only
took 4 lymph nodes out when he discovered they did not
carry any cancer cells, and that's why I do not qualify for the
trials. Apparently you need to have had 6 taken out! Now I
find out that if I hadn't delayed, I could have been onto my
second cycle of chemo as we speak!

The thing that distresses me most is that I wasn't told I didn't
qualify, with only 4 nodes removed, for the 6 node protocol at
my first meeting in hospital. It is pretty devastating.

The other disappointing issue is that even before I was
diagnosed I had already worked voluntarily with women
who were on clinical trials from all around Australia, so I saw
being on the trials myself as a positive (sorry about that pun)
legacy for future sufferers of breast cancer.

I had also developed a rapport with Kathryn and Annette —
the clinical trials nurses here at the hospital — during the

information sessions before my chemo and radiotherapy. And now they won't be treating me, I feel as though I am out on my own, all by myself. However after seeing me sobbing in the oncology room, Annette and Kathryn have adopted me and have said they will continue to help me even though I'm not a legal triallist. They are so lovely, it affirms my belief in the genuine goodness of people.

Anyway, what's now happening is that basic chemo starts on Friday morning. The good thing is at least now I can confirm my 6 month idyll (oops, oops: I WILL be working very hard) in Greece for the Olympics!

Thanks, FOAMs, for your ongoing love and support. I only hope I live enough decades to repay all your kindnesses.

AM

PS When I'm objective about it, the reason I'm not eligible is that the cancer had not spread enough to taint the nodes. So I will be fine and still live to be that 94-yr-old wicked woman.

Jocelyn Newman's Journey

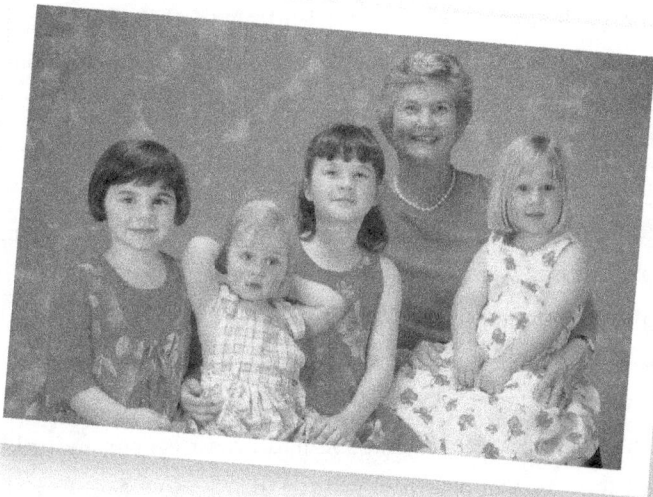

' ... I read about Tamoxifen. Nobody really knew much about
it and I spoke with a young medical scientist at Flinders
University Medical Centre who talked to me over the phone.
He was such a great advocate for this new treatment that I
decided that yes, that's what I'd do.'

*J*ocelyn Newman AO is in Queensland for the Easter school holidays, visiting her son Campbell, Brisbane's Lord Mayor, and spending precious time with her two granddaughters and their mum, Lisa. She is relaxed, carefree and at peace with the world — a far cry from the tumultuous times in 1993 and 1994 when Jocelyn faced not one but two bouts of cancer within six months.

'In 1993, I was a fairly new Tasmanian Senator in the Australian Parliament. I was happily married, with two adult children, when I was diagnosed with uterine cancer. Fortunately, this was caught in time and after a hysterectomy I recovered and was ready to get back to work,' says Jocelyn. 'At the time I admit to thinking to myself, "How do I deal with that?" But it was okay and I got on with life.'

Within six months Jocelyn had what she calls 'my second warning'.

'Funnily enough, looking back, what I remember about being diagnosed with breast cancer was the press conference I did in Parliament House. It was one of those Sunday ones, ready for the Monday papers, and it was one of the hardest things I have ever done in my life,' she says.

She was now a Shadow Minister under Liberal leader John Hewson and she announced that she had breast cancer and told the public that she was stepping down from the Shadow Ministry. 'I just can't give my all to fighting the disease and staying on in Parliament and honourably doing the job of Shadow Minister.'

The timing was not good. The following Monday, a significant Liberal Party meeting was held and Jocelyn hoped that 'the solemnity of my announcement and the seriousness of the disease I was fighting' would help unify the factional fighting within the party under a stable leadership. 'Sadly, that didn't happen,' she adds.

Jocelyn always had regular mammograms and it was during a time between these when she felt the lump in her left breast. It was quickly diagnosed as a tumour. 'Years previously, I had also detected a small lump, had it tested and it was found to be just a calcified spot. But blow me down if this cancer wasn't in exactly that same spot.

'When they confirmed it was cancer I went cold, my brain froze and, coming on top of the other cancer, I did feel I'd had a hard run,' she confesses.

Jocelyn wasn't entirely surprised at being diagnosed with breast cancer. Both her mother and her grandmother and, she has since discovered, other family members had breast cancer. 'So it was something that you almost expected but you hoped to God that it wouldn't happen. However, none of my family have ever died from the disease so that gives me hope.'

Nevertheless, this doesn't mean that Jocelyn doesn't worry for her daughter and her four granddaughters. 'We specialise in women in our family,' she jokes, 'so it is an ongoing concern. I also know that my son could be at risk, because it isn't widely known that men also get this disease.'

As a consequence of her public profile, Jocelyn received hundreds of letters of support from all around Australia. 'But really the saddest letters were from the men who felt that there was little recognition or support for men with breast cancer. Many of them felt very uncomfortable about getting help.'

After standing down in Canberra, Jocelyn returned to Tasmania and 'went through the mill'.

She had a mastectomy — 'Off with her head!' she jokes, — and full axillary clearance, which resulted in lymphoedema in her arm. She shrugs and says, 'The same problem is in my leg from the previous cancer. So now I have enough, thank you! I wear trousers and I have to keep moving.

'Even when I returned to Parliament I used to sit back in my seat and do arm stretching exercises for much of the day — just like the blokes sitting back in their chairs. No one knew until I retired and then I told them what I'd been doing!' she laughs.

In many ways Jocelyn's uterine cancer overshadowed her breast cancer diagnosis. When she had a hysterectomy, the family gathered quickly. Jocelyn recalls bursting into tears and sobbing, 'I feel so mutilated, so mutilated.' Then, when she was faced with a mastectomy, she and her family were extremely worried about how they would cope with this second 'mutilation'.

'I am sure the mastectomy was the sensible thing to do, but nowadays, with lumpectomies the go, I wouldn't have had to have it. I do envy people these days who still have two breasts.'

Yet she still feels intense disappointment that the surgeon would not do a double mastectomy. 'With my family history, I pleaded with my surgeon to do a double mastectomy. Being flat-chested was no big deal. Being lopsided was a horrible look. I think he was a man who expected women to have breasts. His attitude was: if this breast hasn't had cancer in it — yet — then we can't take it off.' But I would have preferred to have been flat-chested. That would have been simple, cheap and 'no worries'.

Once she'd recovered from her surgery, Jocelyn was advised by oncologists to go through chemotherapy. She thought it seemed very daunting and too demanding, and self-deprecatingly says, 'I was gutless; I was looking for an easy option.'

She had already told her doctors categorically that — having had traumatic experiences during her uterine cancer treatments — radiotherapy was not an alternative. 'I didn't like those options. Can I have another menu please?' she had asked.

Although she knew what she didn't want, she had no idea what other choices were available for her.

'At the very time I was lying in hospital in Launceston, the Federal Parliament was having an inquiry into breast cancer. I contacted Trish Worth, a colleague of mine in the House of Reps, and asked her to let me know who the most impressive witnesses were, and what was the best evidence of treatment. So daily, as they came off the press, I read all the transcripts and I read about Tamoxifen. Nobody really knew much about it. I spoke with a young medical scientist at Flinders University Medical Centre who talked to me over the phone. He was such a great advocate for this new treatment that I decided that yes, that's what I'd do.'

Tamoxifen was new in those days and although her doctors

were not adverse to that as the only treatment, they didn't want to be responsible should things go wrong. Jocelyn took control of her health and said, 'No — that's what I want!'

'Some people thought I was crazy — because it was new and because I didn't have any other treatments. But I have never been sorry. Maybe, looking back, I may have wondered if I was being "a little too smart by half" and thought, "Will I be sorry?"'

When Jocelyn went for her five-year check-up, she asked to remain on the drug for another two years. 'This was the lucky charm in my pocket,' she grins. Even now she follows all of the new and exciting advances in medication and inside thinks to herself, 'There go I.'

When I ask how her family and friends coped with her breast cancer diagnosis, she candidly answers, 'I have no idea — I really haven't. My husband was wonderful. I was treated beautifully by him. He ran the home, did the cooking, but because he had retired he was already doing much of that. As I was a Minister in Parliament, he kept the home going while I was away in Canberra and so, with my diagnosis, nothing much changed.

'The children had left home at the time and although they didn't immediately fly back to Tasmania to my bedside, they are, and were during that time, very good rocks to stand on,' she says proudly. On reflection, and prompted by her daughter-in-law, Jocelyn recalls the family did come down to make sure she was coping — 'But they'd done it once before and, for us all, the breast cancer wasn't nearly as scary. They'd already been through everything! We're a phlegmatic family really, aren't we?'

Whilst friends are often the cornerstone of emotional support during times of illness, Jocelyn explains that her situation was unusual and different from most. As an army wife, she had lived in many different towns and cities, so true friends were scattered all around Australia. Her longtime friends from her early years in Melbourne were compassionate — but not in the same State as her.

She also rationalises that when she moved into Parliament, she met and was friendly with lots and lots of people over the whole of

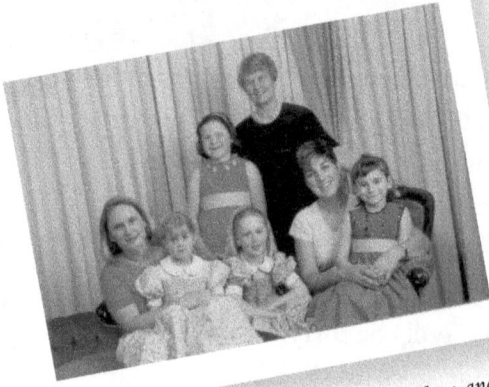

Jocelyn with her daughter and daughter-in-law, and her granddaughters

Tasmania but she didn't have many close friends. 'People do gossip about you. There is no privacy, so you protect yourself by not having too many people who are very close, especially in the home situation. But it wasn't hard because I have such a loving family. We just closed ranks around the wounded bird — that was all I needed.'

She does, however, feel for those who are not so loved and supported. 'I feel deep sympathy for those women who are on their own or become alone when their husbands or partners walk out. I just don't know how they cope.'

She also had enormous public support and felt very touched by the boxes and boxes of letters that people sent her during her illness. 'I have kept them all — that sort of kindness I've never wanted to throw away.'

Nevertheless, Jocelyn is a self-proclaimed independent and dogged person and she knew that if she was to recover, she was the only person who could make it happen. 'For pity sake,' she told herself, 'get home and get on with whatever is left of your life!' And she did.

When asked about how she felt when faced with death and dying, she is thoughtful. After deep consideration, she admits that 'It was too long ago now. So much has happened in my life since then that my emotions back in 1994 have been washed away.

'Having had two serious operations to deal with life-threatening cancers so close together, an awful lot of those thoughts and emotions happened at the time of the first cancer,' she suggests. 'That was my first instance of facing my own mortality and I think after that I had a more pragmatic view with the breast cancer, thinking that I'd been okay then, so let's see what this brings.'

Jocelyn acknowledges that while she doesn't dwell on it, she is more prone to thinking that maybe the breast cancer may return. And she is certainly aware of her own mortality — but in a positive way. 'I just get out and do things now; I don't ask why not, because you are a long time dead.'

And her full life is indeed testimony to that positive attitude.

The period immediately following her recovery from the breast cancer surgery was one of the best times for Jocelyn in her political career. 'I went back to Parliament after a few months, and the new leader of the Opposition, Alexander Downer, asked me to come back on the front bench. I told him I was going to be a little sensible and quietly look after myself. He then said to me, "What if I said it was as Shadow Minister for Defence?" I instantly replied, "Done!"

'That was my dream. I'd been Shadow Minister of the junior portfolio of Defence and had written policies for numerous departments, but this was what I really wanted to do,' she says enthusiastically, then wryly adds, 'When John Howard got into government, he did appoint me as a Minister — but it was for Social Security!'

Almost immediately after her diagnosis, Jocelyn became a stalwart champion in helping those who have been diagnosed with breast cancer. 'Being a Parliamentarian, I found I could use my position to help the cause. So I tried to do what I could when I had the opportunity.'

Since retiring from Federal Parliament, Jocelyn is very active in her support for the Breast Cancer Network of Australia (BCNA). She says her life is filled with good humour and that everything she does with BCNA turns into a laugh. 'We have all had breast cancer and so we are sisters under the skin. It is a very nice feeling when you have a National Conference and we all get together, compare notes and generally have fun.'

As well as finding her work with the Network enjoyable, Jocelyn says it is 'truly inspirational'. She becomes especially emotional when she speaks of the National Field of Women held in Melbourne at the MCG. 'Before the big AFL match we were on the field, helicopters were circling overhead, and all of us — men, women and children — felt such a buzz. Here we were standing in the middle of the MCG in pink, creating a giant pink lady silhouette — getting the message about breast cancer out to not only those at the ground, but to the millions watching TV around the country. It was amazing.

'I couldn't stay after the display and savour the feeling because I had to catch the last plane back to Canberra. So I raced to the airport. I was running down the concourse when a young man stopped me and said, "I rang up and gave money to you guys." Another couple added they, too, had donated, and when I got onto the plane the stewardess told me she'd wanted to go to the MCG but couldn't change her roster. Of course, I was still in my hot-pink poncho! These were three very touching take-outs from that night. I still remember them clearly because it was extremely emotional for everyone — spectators and participants,' she says.

As an advocate for the BCNA, Jocelyn is very proud of the support given to women — all around Australia and beyond. One example she recounts is of being on Norfolk Island and speaking to the CWA group about the Breast Cancer Network and its achievements. 'I told them about meeting a woman in Philadelphia a few months earlier. We got talking and she told me she worked for breast cancer. I told her I did, too, and I shared with her some of our successes here in Australia. I gave her a copy of the *My Journey Kit*. She took that back with her to the US, where the community workers were so impressed with its practical value to women that they were planning to produce a similar kit in America.'

On Breast Cancer Day in 2006, Jocelyn went to the annual remembrance ceremony at the Calvary Hospital in Canberra. She pauses, struggling with her emotions as she remembers the day. 'I sat down beside this lovely young couple with their toddler son. When the speaker was introduced, the young lady got up to speak about her diagnosis with breast cancer. That episode really got to me more than my own cancer. I still feel churned up thinking of that young woman and her very young family and hope that everything is okay.'

Having twice looked death in the face, Jocelyn has kept faith with her maxim of squeezing every ounce out of her life. She recently travelled across the world, spending a month sailing across the seas as a passenger in a container ship. 'After Queensland friends had experienced travelling overseas this way, they urged me on, saying I had the temperament. And so I just had to do it. It took me two years to find a ship going to where I wanted to travel and at the right time. I was the only passenger — indeed, the only woman on board — and then to make it even more interesting, the crew spoke almost no English. All of that contributed to making it such an amazing experience,' she beams.

'That first trip took me from the east coast of America to Cartegena in Colombia, South America then through the Panama Canal across the Pacific to New Zealand and home. I loved it so much I took another trip from Australia through the Suez Canal to the United Kingdom. Then my third container ship took me from Tokyo down the east coast of Asia to Singapore.'

I ask why she travels this way and not enjoying the luxury of cruise ships. Jocelyn says simply, 'The trips are peaceful, not very expensive, and hardly any passengers to bother me! The crews are very nice, the food is simple and there are books, flying fish, birds and denizens of the deep to keep you alert!'

The interview ends, and we walk down the street together. Jocelyn is about to head off on another little adventure — this time with granddaughters in tow — to look over Brisbane city from the newly finished council building. She is relishing the prospect of spending time with her family. Suddenly she stops and tells me, 'Go and talk to some "stars"; I'm just an ex-pollie. Talk to stars whose stories will inspire.'

But to my mind, this petite former senator, who has put the nightmare of cancer behind her and is actively working with breast cancer networks, *is* a star.

Hi FOAMs

One down and only 5 to go!

Chemo was fine — no problems — and Ursula and Annette, my nurses, were so, so kind. I know they gave me lots of protective love mixed in with the nasties so I am going to be fabulous.

Thank you all for your prayers and best wishes; they obviously put a protective coat around me too.

Pete and I are off to the farm for the weekend to revel in the bucolic quietness and normality of life.

Once this is finished, look forward to the party!

AM

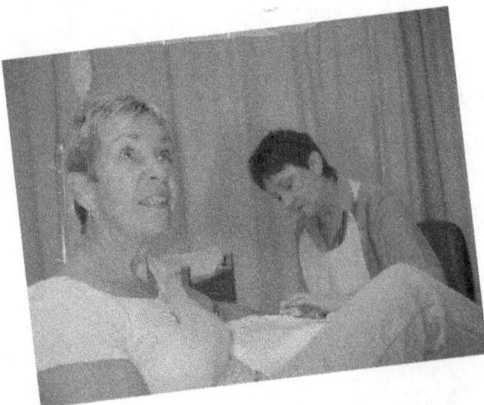

Kate Friis's Journey

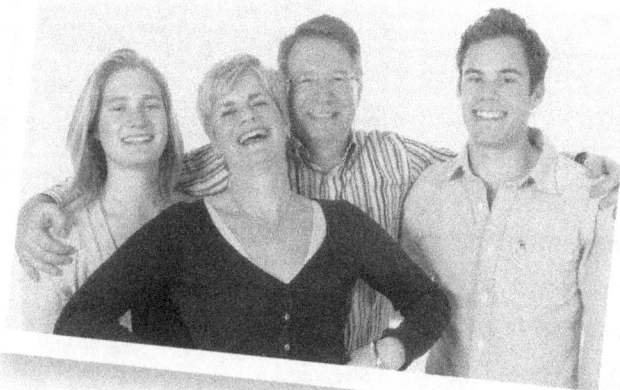

'Whilst that doctor acknowledged that she could never understand fully my fears — of 25 years of worrying that I would get breast cancer — her view clarified my stand and ... on Tuesday 20 November 2007 I made the irreversible decision to have a bilateral mastectomy.'

On a bleak, shivery October day in a windswept Balmain, I escape the blustery rain to chat with Kate Friis. With a cuppa in hand, we start to talk. Instantly I am warm and relaxed.

It is only eight months since Kate made the enormous decision to have a double mastectomy, and while there are still moments of loss she is now adjusting well to post-reconstruction life with her two new 'cherry cupcakes'.

Most women who are diagnosed with breast cancer ask 'How?' or 'Why me?' Kate Friis has lived her whole life not worrying why or how she would get the disease — but when.

'I have known about the history of breast cancer in my family for as long as I can remember. My mum, Kathleen, was diagnosed when I was about three or four and it was already invasive when the doctors found it. She had a radical mastectomy and for the next four years she struggled with the illness. It was gruesome. The cancer went to her bones and to her brain. She was only 42 when she died and I was just eight,' Kate says.

When I ask about her mother during Kate's early years of childhood, a shadow crosses her face, and she tells me that, astonishingly, she doesn't

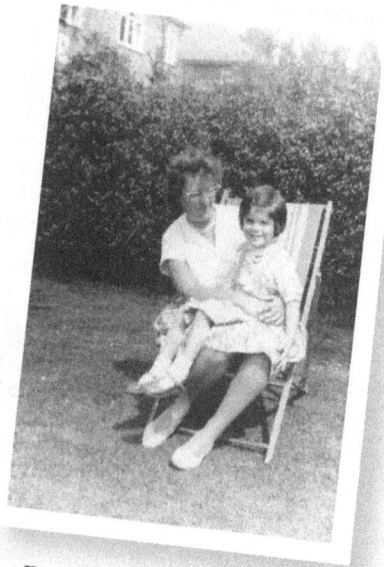

Kate as a child, with her mother

remember anything. 'Not remembering my mum has been my greatest struggle and regret in life.'

Kate is a counsellor and thus understands that young children often shut down as a protection mechanism. She was also the youngest in the family and was not privy to the daily problems of her mother's terminal illness. Because Kate's mother was so ill, she spent a lot of time with her maternal grandmother and was kept away from any of the unpleasantness of her mother's sickness and frail health.

'I appreciate that this is what probably happened to me. I do have a couple of flashes of my mother which I believe are genuine memories, but I really do not have any true recollections.'

Kate thinks that she probably found her calling as a trauma and grief counsellor because of her own personal challenges with loss and grief. 'As a child back 40 years ago, I was very protected and excluded from any sad elements and I lived in a vacuum. I didn't go to my mother's funeral, which in hindsight is such a sad thing. But I know it was well intentioned, and that's what they did in those days. I did sense what was happening, but as the baby in the family I was kind of parked away from the darkness of death.'

Cancer continued to haunt Kate's family. 'When I was 27, my middle sister, who was then 32 and living in the Middle East, got breast cancer. She found a lump and went back to London to have it checked out. Within days she had had a mastectomy, losing her right breast, and all of her lymph nodes were removed. We were also in London, and so my husband and I were her main support until her husband arrived. Obviously, we were very involved with looking after her and all of the trauma surrounding her treatments.

'The absolute terror of breast cancer really hit me at that time. Although I didn't remember Mum's fight with the disease, my sister's diagnosis at such a young age resurrected all of the terror and horror of this cancer. I remember thinking that our whole family would get breast cancer and we were all going to die.'

Until her sister's diagnosis, Kate admits she had lived what is a normal egocentric life, growing up with the usual teenage issues, going off to uni and not really thinking about mortality and what might be.

'I had shut all the fear out but this threw us all back into emotional turmoil. The decision I made this year to have both of my breasts removed is based in my history. I have been worried for 25 years about getting breast cancer — since my sister was diagnosed — and I believed it was our family destiny,' confesses Kate.

The spectre of cancer continued to hover over Kate when, only a few years after her middle sister's diagnosis, her eldest sister was diagnosed with cancer at age 40.

'It was a large tumour on her kidney, and she was living in Australia. I'm English, and we were still living in England at the time so although it wasn't breast cancer, my sister's illness confirmed my fears that our family must have a predisposition to getting cancer. She recovered from that illness, but fast-track another 15 years and that sister was diagnosed with breast cancer. Happily, she has survived.

'Throughout all these years, my fear of getting breast cancer increased and at times became quite debilitating, particularly once I had a family of my own. I would look at my two young children and become almost paralysed with the fear of history repeating itself. I couldn't imagine how the kids would cope if I were to die. I decided my only option was to become incredibly vigilant and so I started having annual breast checks with a breast physician, Ros Cohen, from my late 20s. And then in my late 30s, my paranoia and my sisters' diagnoses made me up the ante and I began having a check-up every six months,' she explains.

Despite her extreme worry during those years, nothing had shown up in any of the scans so it seemed Kate was now the only one of her family to have escaped the haunting diagnosis of breast cancer — but not for long.

During her routine check in March 2007, several small specks showed up on the mammogram of her right breast. 'Because the doctor was concerned, I had a core biopsy, which showed a thickening of the tissue. I was heading off overseas and so of course I was very relieved that it turned out to be benign. But inside me there was a little voice wondering if it could be cancer. So I booked the next set of tests for five months' time,' she explains.

'When I had those scans done in early September the specks were still there and the medical staff had thought they had changed a little. Because the APEC forum was being held in Sydney, I had to wait several extra days for the results, which added to my stress. There was no lump, just the little white specks.

'Interestingly, there were five doctors who looked at the X-rays and three of them gave me the all-clear, but the other two doctors — who were both female, and included my breast physician — expressed concern and wanted me to investigate the specks further through surgery. They were much more cautious, and Dr Cohen actually told me she thought the lumps were benign calcifications, but that it was better to do the lumpectomy and make sure.

'The other doctors really felt very sure the spots were also just calcifications and that surgery wasn't necessary, but I guess they were also cognisant of their liability and so endorsed the surgery. I am not casting any aspersions on the male doctors, but I did wonder if the two women had almost a sixth sense,' she says thoughtfully.

So Kate went into surgery and a lumpectomy was performed with the general opinion that it would not be cancerous. Kate did feel a sense of acceptance that maybe 'this was to be the time I get breast cancer — but of course I hoped it would not be malignant'.

'When James and I were waiting for the histology results, the doctors were still confident it was benign. So when the doctors told me I had a small, high-grade DCIS (ductal carcinoma in situ), they were more surprised than I was. Ironically, from the build-up from the doctors — who had almost suggested that surgery was a waste of time — I had got my head around to thinking that actually this wasn't going to be the time. But it was.

'This was the ultimate irony. For years and years I was always expecting the medical guys to tell me I had breast cancer. Here I was, nearly 50 years old, and I thought I was going to escape. I was almost lulled into this false sense of security.

'When the doctor gave me the bad news, my stomach dropped but I remained very calm on the outside. The surgeon was kind and very matter-of-fact, which I later understood was because it was not an invasive cancer. He told me I was one of the fortunate women who had caught the cancer early. Slightly strange to have the words "fortunate" and "cancer" in the same sentence, isn't it?' she asks me.

'The reality was, though, that I was relieved to know it was classified as an early cancer and it was not invasive. I understood that, but I needed to know more and to be fully aware of everything about my diagnosis, so I did my own research.

'Very quickly I appreciated that DCIS wasn't an immediate risk for me, but the more I read the more I was concerned about the longer-term effects and whether it would eventually spread. I realised that we just don't know what makes a carcinoma in situ break the cell wall and become invasive.'

Kate still had lots of questions, and alarm bells started sounding as she tried to filter through the mountains of information she was gathering. 'Especially worrying for me was when I asked the doctors if I could assume that I wouldn't have a recurrence as neither of my sisters had had one. Their answer was an emphatic "No." They told me I couldn't make this assumption because, although we are related, our cancers were quite different.'

The doctors treating Kate were, however, very confident that they had clear margins around the tumour and said that all that was required was a six-week course of radiotherapy and a five-year course of Tamoxifen.

However, this treatment recommendation caused some confusion for Kate. 'Here I am hearing that the diagnosis is a pre-cancer growth, but yet the doctors are treating it as if it is a cancer. They said that they treat the two types exactly the same, which at the time I thought was odd but I accepted it.

'The doctors said I should start radiotherapy in November. I went for the first meeting with the doctors and asked hundreds of questions so I felt I had a complete grasp of what was happening to me. On the second visit, with my husband, Dr Cohen asked me had I ever considered having bilateral prophylactic mastectomies,' says Kate.

'I was a little surprised and I asked her, "Do you mean having both of my breasts removed?" I had never even considered that option. But

I had absolutely total respect for her and it was really only because she had raised it as a possibility that I felt I needed to consider that option.'

The suggestion — not that she should *do* it, but that she should *consider* it — started the whole three-month research project during which Kate looked at all options to determine whether this was the right choice for her.

During those three months, Kate went through a complete shift — from a position of 99 per cent rejection of the double mastectomy idea to a belief that this would be the best path for her to travel. The decision wasn't very simple or easy and she admits to 'having several melt-downs in that period' and feeling that it 'was all just too hard to get my head around'.

'I kept thinking that Dr Cohen had planted the suggestion for a reason and because I trusted her implicitly I decided to look into the idea. I went to a plastic surgeon for further information and continued to do an enormous amount of investigation.

'Making the decision was the hardest thing to do — without a shadow of a doubt. If I decided to go the "full monty" and have both breasts removed, there was no going back. The emotional stress was really overwhelming for me at times. I needed time to make the decision, but I also knew that I could not put off treatment for very long.'

Kate felt confident there was no risk in the short term. She had absolute assurances from her medical team that the lumpectomy had been a success and there would be no risks for her in deferring her radiotherapy until January 2008. She knew that irradiated tissue was very difficult to work with so her window of opportunity in which to make a decision was only three months long.

'Feeling pressured with all of these options and choices in my head, I went and talked it through with my GP. She told me she felt I had as much information and knowledge about the alternatives as she did. She told me I just had to make the decision and gave me two very valuable bits of advice to stop me going mad.'

The first recommendation was that Kate set a date for her decision. The other suggestion was to get a second and different viewpoint. At the time, Kate was talking to lots of people, but they were all from the same cancer care unit and so had very similar mind sets.

'I listened to what she said and I did! I chose 20 November — a week before my 50th birthday — as the date I would make my final decision.

'I then went to see a respected breast cancer oncologist, who couldn't understand why I would consider going down this radical route. She told me it was too extreme, much harder on my body than any medication and too invasive. She told me there was nothing to fear from radiation, nothing to fear about taking Tamoxifen. And although she didn't use these words, she felt I was taking a sledgehammer approach to my recovery. She told me that if she was in my position she would not have surgery. She said she was very worried about the dangers of the long time I would be under anaesthetics.'

Kate came out of the consultation a little shell-shocked, but now declares it was the best thing that could have happened. 'The opposite view made me really look and think about what I really wanted to do with my body.

'Whilst that doctor acknowledged that she could never understand fully my fears — of 25 years of worrying that I would get breast cancer — her view clarified my stand and I am very grateful to her for her honesty,' says Kate warmly.

'So on Tuesday, 20 November 2007 I made the irreversible decision to have a bilateral mastectomy. Once the decision was made, I rang the plastic surgeon, who booked me in for 15 February 2008. This seemed like a long way ahead — I would have loved to have done it sooner, but I was very fortunate to get that date.

'Still, I had niggles of worry about whether I was doing the right thing. I worried that maybe it was too much. However, during this time the support and encouragement of my husband and kids was constant. James never interfered in my decision-making and would only say repeatedly that all he cared about was having me around for as long as possible so we could grow old together.

'My son, Ben, was always supportive, too. When I needed to talk, he never tired of helping me grapple with the complexities of the huge decision I was trying to make. On one of the frequent occasions when I was agonising about what to do, he hugged me tightly and said, "Mum, you know we will support whatever decision you make, but once you've made your mind up, you must back yourself." Wise words. Little did I realise how important his advice would be over the following months. And that message guided me whenever I felt any doubts creeping in.'

Kate is very proud of her family's involvement in her decision and is quick to emphasise that their support was constant and unreserved. Without that unconditional love, she says she would never have been able to come through with the strength she has.

At the time of her diagnosis, her daughter, Hanne, was overseas in England on her gap year. Kate explains, 'We had always promised her that if anything happened when she was overseas we would tell her immediately. I needed to tell her from the start about the test. I couldn't just have James ring and tell her, "Oh, by the way Mum has cancer and has just had a lumpectomy!" We needed to prepare her. But as she was 12,000 miles [20,000 km] away, Hanne was understandably very scared and tense. She waited up all night by the phone for news on the day when I went in for the test results.

'We weren't really prepared ourselves for the cancer diagnosis and so it was very hard for James to have to tell Hanne. Because we hadn't expected the cancer diagnosis we were also raw and Hanne felt that fear and she was devastated. She cried the whole night long — it was so hard on her being by herself so far away,' recalls Kate emotionally. 'Hanne wanted to fly home immediately to be at my side and be there for me. But we tried to reassure her that there was no need.

'We played it down, stressing it was a very early cancer. But she was hearing the news and reacting through memories of her grandmother dying so young of this deadly disease. And no matter how many times I told her I was not about to die, this seemed a death sentence for her.

'She was also very protective of me and didn't let me know how badly she took the news. Thank goodness I didn't know, because I'm not sure I could have handled the grief and concerns of my little girl so far away from home.

'I tried to convince her I was fine, that I didn't look any different, and that I was coping fine. But my husband pulled me up, saying, "What are we doing to her? Hanne has a real need to come back to the family and make sure for our sakes, but importantly for her own sake, that everything is fine. Let her come."'

So Hanne returned to Australia. 'I know there was no medical reason for her to come back and interrupt her gap year, but she insisted she wanted to be at home with the family. She wanted to be supportive of me. And that is what is special about families: they gather together for strength. She was home for two weeks. This was also a wonderful time for me — and for us as a family. Once Hanne saw that things were going to be okay she was happy to go back to England.'

To compound the impact of Kate's diagnosis was the almost simultaneous breast cancer diagnosis of someone in Kate and James's inner circle. 'Within two weeks, both James and his business partner of 16 years had to face the fact that both of their wives had breast cancer,' explains Kate, still amazed at the freakish coincidence.

Kate and the family had planned a holiday that summer of 2008 and together they made a decision that they would still enjoy a trip to New York and then return to Australia ready to prepare for Kate's surgery in February.

'One of the most purposeful decisions I made was to get myself very fit and healthy so I would get through the operation in the best possible shape. I also spent a lot of time thinking about my new body — how the new breasts would look — so that I was prepared both physically and emotionally.'

The day before the operation was a Friis family day and they went bowling and to Fox studios and just enjoyed what Kate calls 'the simple family day of fun'.

As the morning of 15 February dawned, Kate recalls feeling 'as calm as a cucumber. I had slept well and I was ready — which is quite amazing. Although I knew I had made the right decision to have the operation, I was absolutely terrified of the anaesthesia not working. I have a great fear of being awake during surgery.

'I was lying ready to go into the operating room and I got into a panic. I told myself I had to calm down and deal with this. So I envisaged all my family and my friends, my army of supporters, in the space around me, knowing that they were loving me and looking after me. I looked into every face and was calmed.

'I was then wheeled into the operating theatre and the plastic surgeon started measuring me up. As he leaned over he said to me, "It's not too late to call it all off. I could be at golf!" But of course there was no turning back and I knew I had to go forward and just do it.'

The operation to remove Kate's breasts and to reconstruct her new breasts took 12 hours. 'I went in with breasts and I came out with new breasts. However, the operation had taken a little longer as the micro-surgery hadn't quite taken in the beginning. But ultimately, everything was fine.

'The first 48 hours after the reconstruction operation was difficult as I was pretty doped up and the wounds were checked every 20 minutes to ensure the blood supply to my new breasts was flowing and the grafts were taking. But the relief I felt about the whole thing being over was euphoric. And the euphoria built and built. Perhaps the morphine had something to do with that!' she adds.

'I was alive. And despite feeling like I had been run over by a truck, and being in a lot of pain, I had a genuine sense of relief and satisfaction that I had done it. Then the second day I had a terrible time. The pain was dreadful and I started doubting I'd done the right thing. So I told myself to be logical and to think about the reasons I had done it.

'My training as a counsellor certainly helped me think it all through. But there is really no psychological preparation, so I had to do it all by myself — for myself. And I did,' she says with pride.

'And the truth is, I was ecstatic! I wanted to tell the world. I was on such a sustained high, which continually reinforced my conviction that my decision to have the double mastectomy was the right one.

'During the 11 days I spent in hospital I set myself all kinds of crazy goals. I wanted to recover as quickly as possible, so I mapped out a 1 kilometre route around the wards, which I walked several times a day, carrying my six drips in two pillowcases.

'I also decided I'd write a book and so madly started scribbling notes on the backs of envelopes and any bits of paper I could get my hands on. I even imagined myself at my book launch and being interviewed on TV wearing a plunging neckline to show off my new boobs to the rest of the world. Thankfully, much to everyone's relief, I calmed down — but it took two weeks!' she laughs.

Kate remembers clearly the first time she saw her new chest — five days after the operation. 'I had wanted to unwrap the bandages by myself — sort of a personal discovery — but my husband had come up and so it was more a public showing,' she chuckles. 'It took almost a day until I could really look. I remember saying, "If this is the best I will look, then that's okay."

'Of course, I do have fleeting thoughts about whether I did the right thing, but belonging to a family with a history like mine, I am very confident it was the right decision. Neither of my sisters has had a double mastectomy and they are fine, so maybe I was a little over-reactive. But the reality for me is that it is pretty clear this is the best course and in the future years I can look back and have no regrets.'

It is only natural for our minds to wander over the 'What ifs' and even a woman as strongly decisive as Kate admits to a bit of an emotional rollercoaster ride.

'Thankfully, I am more or less back on track. At times, the loss of my breasts and the fear of what might have been, creeps up and taps me on the shoulder when I am least expecting it. Before I know it

I am down at the bottom of the emotional seesaw. The good news is that I know it is only temporary and that I'll bounce back and squeeze every bit of joy and fun out of my life,' she declares.

With her family's history of breast cancer hanging over Kate's whole life — and being the defining reason for her brave decision to endure a radical double mastectomy — genetic testing was something that almost taunted Kate.

'I wasn't too sure about getting genetic tests done. I had considered having the test about 10 years ago but decided against it because I believed that a positive result might somehow make getting breast cancer a self-fulfilling prophecy. And back then I wasn't prepared to consider removing my healthy breasts as a purely preventative measure,' explains Kate.

'But when I was diagnosed with breast cancer, albeit early and small, it was completely different and I started to think that if I tested positive for one of the two known gene mutations, it would make surgery a much more logical and sensible option.

'So one of my sisters and I had the test and when we went to get the results, we were shocked to learn that we tested negative. We presumed at least one of us would be positive so although I was relieved, it made me more confused about making decisions to have my surgery. Nevertheless, even though I don't have those genes, I know I did the best thing for me and I have absolutely no fear of the future,' adds Kate with quiet confidence.

With hindsight, Kate is also grateful that she didn't opt to have the tests earlier. 'There are serious implications to genetic testing. For example, if I had taken the test 10 years ago, I wonder — with that negative result — if I would have been as vigilant.'

Kate has a happy and gregarious personality and when questioned about the lighter side of her journey with breast cancer, she laughs about the situation that her plastic surgeon faced when constructing her new breasts. 'I'd put on a lot of weight several years earlier. I had been in a very stressful job, including working with survivors of the Bali bombings. I realised I was not healthy and over the following two years I had deliberately, and delightedly I might add, lost a lot of weight through a serious diet and exercise regime.

'When the doctor was assessing me a few months before my surgery, he said, "Well, you are a C cup now but you don't have much fat so we'll be lucky to get you a B cup." I then asked was there anything I could do, like putting on weight. He thought I'd not be able to make any real difference in the coming two months — but you haven't seen me eat! So I piled on 5 kilos over Christmas and enough went to my tummy so that when the doctor took fat from my stomach to make my boobs, I did get a slightly larger cup size!'

She also recalls the quintessential moment that seems to sum up her journey with breast cancer. 'When I was contemplating breast reconstruction, my adorable friend Andrea suggested it might help if I thought of my new breasts as friends rather than imposters. So as soon as I decided to go ahead with surgery she began referring to them as my "cherry cupcakes". When she visited me in hospital a couple of days after the operation she arrived doubled up with laughter and carrying a small cake box. Inside were two barely recognisable cupcakes that she had accidentally dropped on the floor as she got out of the hospital lift. She squashed them back together and proudly presented me with two "reconstructed cherry cupcakes"!' Kate laughs loudly, then adds, 'Well — that's Kate now — reconstructed and sweet.'

Kate is now reconciled with herself, with her new 'cherry cupcakes', and comfortable about her very radical decision.

'Basically, it came down to taking a decision that I would never regret and one that would give me peace of mind. I'd lived for 25 years with the fear of getting breast cancer, and the choice I made took away that fear once and for all.'

From: AnneMarie
Subject: CHEMO 2 — YUK
Sent: 6 July 2003

Hi Wonderful FOAMs

It's Sunday morning.

Well, I thought that I was a pretty strong woman throughout
my life so far, but suddenly I was called upon to exert even
more strength than I ever knew I had.

I saw my oncologist on Friday morning, all psyched up for
another dose of chemo. I'd done it easy the first time and all
I thought it took was a strong and positive mind. Doc was
shocked I still had my hair — only one of a couple of people
on my heavy dose of chemo who survive the first two weeks!
See, I knew I was doing well and a tough gal! Although I have
to admit to now being a little like a shaggy dog, dropping
hairs wherever I go. Now if only I can hang on until my
Versace lunch on Friday I'll be very happy!

When I went in for my chemo dose the nurse struggled to
find a vein to insert the drain line into. After four unsuccessful
stabbings she finally got a vein to take. I may now have to
move to a port cut into my chest. Oh well, that may be better
than a blackened hand!!!

The chemo then went well ... so well I went off to do the grocery
shopping. This was a new experience, as Pete always does it!

I came home for a rest when a terrible wave of nausea hit
me. After successfully making the bowl I lay down for a bit of

a sleep to recover. But all afternoon the waves kept coming until I'd nothing left to vomit. After talking with the doc I was admitted to hospital. Even there with drips and injections, they still struggled to keep anything down. I was exhausted by the constant vomiting and heaving — both emotionally and physically. By Saturday lunchtime however, it was finally under control and I came home that afternoon.

This morning everything is a lot better although the aroma of Pete's bacon and eggs sent me scurrying for the balcony!!! And you all know how I love food. It isn't that tempting at the moment, I've got to admit.

This chemo was a real bummer. It is pretty daunting stuff. But that's where the positive attitude comes in. I can either crawl back into bed (tempting!) or go on realising that I will come through the other end and that I can then be proud of myself.

I see it as the challenge of my life, for my life. And by appreciating that I am worth fighting for, it makes carrying the positive attitude easier! Enough indulgence, although I am lucky to have beautiful friends who allow me that.

The next time most of you see me it will be with a beautifully shiny pate. Hey, the bald eagle is me now ... except for those cool days when my collection of bandannas and hats and beanies will be great!

Thank you all for your individual support — in the special phone calls, visits, gifts, flowers, prayers and emails. I am humbled by your caring. Thank you.

Keep smiling ... I still am!

AM

Janelle Gamble's Journey

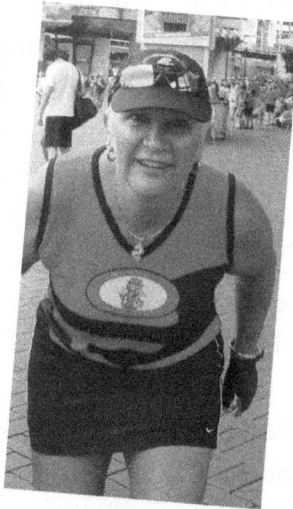

'Dr John told me I had low-grade DCIS — ductal carcinoma in situ — and that I would need a lumpectomy with perhaps some radiotherapy. Fortunately, no mention was made of chemotherapy. At the time I was relieved but now, with hindsight, I wonder if my life would have been different if I had had the chemotherapy.'

Trying to arrange accommodation in Caloundra for a family holiday during September 2007 was proving impossible. When I asked the booking agent why everything was booked out, she said, 'There's some world championships in paddling. It seems to be a big thing, with people coming from every corner of the world.' A big thing indeed — this was the Abreast in Australia 2007 Dragon Boat Regatta. Here, nearly 2000 women who had gone through breast cancer would be paddling in an international carnival celebrating life in the pink.

Now here I am talking with Janelle Gamble, the dynamo behind the event, and a co-founder of Dragons Abreast. Her eyes shine when she talks about how the Abreast in Australia 2007 Dragon Boat Regatta grew from humble beginnings only nine years ago.

In 1998 the first ever conference for women who'd had breast cancer was held in Melbourne, and the Breast Cancer Network was born, with Janelle as Queensland's founding delegate. 'At the conference we heard from a Canadian woman about a dragon boat experiment conducted by a doctor to help rehabilitation after breast cancer. Other delegates Michelle Hatton (NT) and Anna Wellings Booth (ACT) were similarly inspired, and we each formed dragon boat teams of breast cancer survivors,' says Janelle.

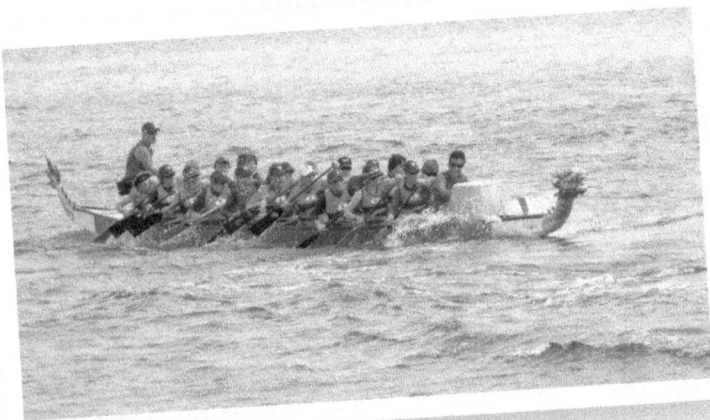

Janelle and fellow team members dragon boat racing

'Then in 2000 Michelle gathered a representative team together and, resplendent in hot pink shirts, we entered the National Dragon Boat Titles in Sydney, calling ourselves the Dragons Abreast team. Problem was we had no paddles, no experience — nothing! We trained by sitting on the bank at Penrith pretending we were in a boat paddling — trying to get some timing going.

'In that regatta there were three boats in our race, and we came a very distant third. But the whole grandstand applauded and we felt fantastic. And that was the start of it for me. I've been committed to the wonderful life of Dragons Abreast ever since.

'Because we are totally inclusive, anyone — even those with no experience — can come along and paddle with us. But if you want to be competitive, there are international regattas. I've been around the world and paddled with amazing women.'

Had she not had breast cancer, Janelle would never have paddled in a dragon boat: 'I hate the water, I am terrified of it, and yet I just love the sport. It is *me* time. I can be what I want to be; there are no expectations other than what I want there to be for myself.'

In explaining the benefits of Dragons Abreast, Janelle is enthusiastic almost to the point of becoming evangelical. 'It fills an important gap for us. Once women finish treatment, they are considered well by the medical profession, who spit us out. We are then on our own and very alone. That's where Dragons Abreast comes in. It picks up those people, gives them a reason to be alive and — because, with cancer, the body had let them down — they can now become physically active, with no expectations or demands. I also think that doing something physical takes away mental pain.'

Like most women diagnosed with breast cancer, Janelle knew almost nothing about the disease that would change her life except that 'Only old ladies got it.' Being fit, with no family history of the disease, and only 40 years old, breast cancer was not on her radar. So she wasn't prepared at all for her first diagnosis. But to have the cancer return twice more has really tested her fire and resilience.

Back in 1991 Janelle noticed a small indentation like a thumbprint on her left breast and went to her GP, who didn't suspect anything was wrong but did suggest a mammogram. 'I went off to the Wesley Hospital and found I was a "lucky one" who'd hit the jackpot!

'I was told things didn't look good and that the doctor would be in touch. They offered to drive me home, but being Miss Independent, I told them I was fine. They did think it was strange that I wasn't upset at all — but I got as far as the car park and totally dissolved. I can't remember driving home.'

Janelle had gone for the test by herself. 'I didn't need any help. I am a very strong woman. I thought I could handle anything.' She also can't recall how she was officially told of the diagnosis. 'All I know is that I went to see Professor John McCaffrey, who was working with the Cancer Council.

'Dr John told me I had low-grade DCIS — ductal carcinoma in situ — and that I would need a lumpectomy with perhaps some radiotherapy. Fortunately, no mention was made of chemotherapy. At the time I was relieved but now with hindsight I wonder if my life would have been different if I had had the chemotherapy.'

At that stage, Janelle's two sons were aged six and eight, and her daughter was a teenager. Husband Blair suspected something was wrong, but his fears were confirmed when 'I just blurted out, "I've got breast cancer and I'm going to die!" "Poor me", "Why me?" — all those despairs that splash through your head.

'I just could not believe that someone as healthy as I was could have an old ladies' disease like breast cancer. It was such a shock. Although 40 is very young, I realised that I was actually very lucky. I'd had my three children. It was just such a shock to me and to everyone. I couldn't believe it and I kept looking at myself and thinking, "I'm so well!"

'My friends were great. They are really quirky! They're not the sort to sympathise and say, "Poor Possum". They told me to get over it! One of my friends brought in a bonsai tree — it was lopsided like I was going to be,' Janelle chuckles.

Janelle is a very practical person and, having accepted her situation, she decided that she just had to get on with it. 'I talked with Professor McCaffrey — such a calm, caring man — and he patiently answered all my questions, almost as if I was the only women ever diagnosed. But there was an urgency to get that lump out of me.'

A lumpectomy was scheduled for that week. However, the biopsy taken after the surgery revealed that there hadn't been completely healthy tissue surrounding the site of the surgery so Janelle was back in theatre within the week, and finally the margins around the tumour site were clear.

She was offered radiotherapy treatment and was told there was no need to have chemotherapy. 'That was the best available treatment at the time. With hindsight, had I had chemo then, the cancer may not have recurred — I really don't know. At the time, I wasn't nervous about not doing chemo; I was absolutely thrilled to not have to go through it.'

When she was in hospital Janelle was offered a support visitor, but of course, once again displaying her independent nature, she told them she was fine: 'The cancer's gone and I don't need anyone up here teaching me how to knit — just keep out of my face!'

The radiotherapy was exhausting for Janelle; she was working as a teacher full-time, looking after two active young boys under nine and trudging up to the hospital each day. 'It was a hard slog. At 40, I was too young to be tired. I was out there doing things, so that did hit me a bit.'

The worst effect of the cancer this first time round was the impact it had on those around her. Whilst most of Janelle's friends stuck by her, she was devastated and is still greatly saddened by the loss of contact with 'my bridesmaid. I tried many times to contact her, but it was like I had a contagious disease, and to this day I've heard nothing from her — not a single word. That really hurts.

'The other thing that really bothered me was that my daughter, Tara, was totally lacking in support — like most other 18-year-olds would have been. It's probably how teenagers cope. She ran away from home and did her own thing. She didn't know what to do or how to handle it. She finally came back but announced she was leaving for overseas in three weeks. She was away in London for about three years. During that time there were lots of phone calls, conversations and growing up. She came back my very best friend in the world. But at the time that was very hard for me to cope with.'

Life went back to normality and apart from regular check-ups, 'I went out and had a good time — leaving cancer behind.' However, she does admit that there is always the fear of cancer in the back of her mind: 'You are never cured. Every ache could be secondaries in my bones; each time I got a cold or a sniffle I'd think, "Oh, it's back!"

'Professor McCaffrey suggested — no, he insisted — that I become a volunteer with the Cancer Council, even though I assured him I was not the volunteer type. But I did the training and worked with women in a similar position to myself; since I had been treated with only radiotherapy and Tamoxifen, I was not equipped to offer peer support to anyone on chemotherapy. Really, this is the most rewarding thing I've done in my life. What is most satisfying is being able to take the fear away from others and therefore myself. I found that peer support has enormous benefit to women who have breast cancer — just being able to say, "I've been there" and understand. It's also being able to offer the practical hints — like always wearing separates to radiation therapy, so you aren't out there lying in just your knickers.'

Then seven years later, almost to the day, Janelle had her routine mammogram at Chermside BreastScreen. Fortunately, John McCaffrey was there at the time and on reading the films told Janelle he didn't like the look of them. Initially, they thought the problem lay in the use of a new brand of film but a second investigation showed that a new cancer had formed in the scar tissue of the original tumour.

'I was all tarted up to go to lunch and champagne with the girls at the Sheraton. I thought, "I am tough, I can deal with this," and walked into the hotel and dissolved,' she says shaking her head. 'This just can't happen a second time — double jeopardy.'

She was annoyed. 'It was so damned inconvenient. My husband and I had planned an overseas holiday. But Blair, ever practical, explained we could always go on a holiday later; now let's get well.'

She again headed into surgery for a further lumpectomy. 'The first scar had healed so well it was invisible. This time they had to take quite a bit more so I ended up looking like my bonsai tree — lopsided!' She chuckles and adds, 'Which I killed purposely.'

Because she couldn't have radiotherapy twice on the same place, Janelle was put on Tamoxifen, the wonder drug of the time. But after 18 months of being 'the complete bitch from hell', gaining weight, and going through mood swings, Janelle threw the tablets away, confident she was healed and had finished with cancer for ever and ever.

'You never, never get cancer three times,' she had said confidently — at the time.

Incredibly, almost seven years to the day once more, Janelle found herself having the regular mammogram in 2004 and facing a third bout of breast cancer.

'I was in total disbelief. Worst of all was that Dr John had died and I didn't know who to turn to professionally — his shoes were too big to fill.'

Again, the diagnosis was very inconvenient. Janelle was packed and ready to travel to Shanghai to compete in the World Dragon Boat Championships. Knowing that this third tumour in the same breast meant a mastectomy, she made the decision to have an interim lumpectomy and then deal with losing her breast when she returned to Australia.

'Within three weeks I was in the boat, competed in the Championships and came straight home into hospital for a mastectomy and immediate reconstruction. I had a good medical team and really felt like I was okay,' she says.

This time round Janelle had chemotherapy. 'I was absolutely dreading it. I did everything possible to avoid it; I just couldn't bear it. When I had been doing peer support visiting, I'd met several women who had been treated with the various forms of chemotherapy, and was aware of how these drugs affected the patients — nausea, hair loss etc — so I *thought* I knew how difficult it was going to be. And that made me scared enough, but in fact I had no idea.

'The first treatment was scary — the unknown — waiting for the needle to deliver its lethal cocktail of drugs. The saline wasn't too bad, but then comes the chill as the real deal snakes through your vein. And it takes so long, sitting there — hooked up to a hubbly bubbly pipe but not nearly as much fun. Finally, that first session was over. But worse was to come: there were six sessions to endure over the following months.'

After the first session of chemotherapy, Janelle decided she was not going back. 'It had all run late; there was a meal of tripe waiting for me in the hospital room, with three other sick ladies — so I threw a tizzy fit and went home to die quietly.

'I didn't want to talk to anyone; I was so pathetic I just lay in bed for days, waiting to die. I was in complete shock about how hard it truly was. I decided I was never doing this again: "No matter how sick I get, I am not doing this again," I vowed.

'It was only my close friend, Leonie, who got me through. I wouldn't let Blair come with me and see me vulnerable. I tell you, she was amazing. It was only at Leonie's insistence that I completed my cycles. There is no way I could be that strong and do that for someone.'

But, of course, she eventually found the strength and battled on.

Janelle acknowledges that her emotional reaction was extreme. She was used to being healthy; feeling nauseous and constantly vomiting was alien and really threw her. 'The first three days after the treatment were always difficult — waves of nausea and feeling like a limp rag doll. As the days passed, so did the nausea, until after three weeks, my strength would return, and I had to mentally prepare for the next session of treatment.'

So negative was her experience of chemotherapy, especially with the red chemo drug Epirubican, that even to this day Janelle gets the trembles every time she sees red cordial or anything bright red. 'Chemo was the worst part of my cancer journey, but I learned how strong women can be and I have found new respect for those who have done this before me.'

So after three bouts of breast cancer, how did she cope? 'I reckon I have coped very well. I don't dwell on it and I focus on things that are important to me, like my family. Now I am about to be a grandmother for the first time — that's important,' she says with a huge grin.

Breast cancer doesn't intrude into Janelle's life at all on a daily basis. But she does admit that it is never going to be far from the back of her mind, especially when women she knows lose the battle. 'We have several ladies in our dragon boat who have secondaries and they are so determined to live every day to the fullest that they are out there, even if they feel lousy, because paddling takes the focus away from their fears. That sort of courage keeps me going to Dragons Abreast.'

When I ask her if there was one secret for getting on with life after cancer, Janelle replies, 'Without wishing to sound selfish, take each day as it comes, have some long-term flexible goals that are within reach and then go for it!'

Whilst Janelle managed her emotions quite well during her cancer journey, she says her children, especially the boys, have had to deal afresh with each new diagnosis. She says, 'They probably know as much as anyone about the disease because they've lived with it — it's all they know. In a positive sense it has given them a compassionate outlook on life.'

She recalls a poignant moment on the day her hair started to fall out after chemotherapy during her last bout of cancer. 'Callum, my youngest, is a motorbike fanatic: bikes are his life, and he is really the tough blokey type. This particular day he noticed after my shower that my hair was shedding everywhere. We sat together and cried. Then he got up and carefully shaved my head. Breast Cancer has really developed a strong bond between us.'

After a cancer diagnosis, death and depression may hover in the subconscious, but Janelle is a shining example of the power of positive energy in overcoming despair.

'You don't have to have cancer to face death. That bus will come along whether you are ready or not — I'm just hoping that my bus is a long way away! And I intend to live my life with no regrets.'

She tells me that she is no longer the person she was before cancer. Although Janelle could never have been described as meek, she has now developed a strength and focus that is born from adversity. 'I know who I am, where I am going and how I am getting there,' she asserts.

Throwing her arms wide she becomes very animated, saying, 'I am really very lucky. My life is full. I travel a lot. I have fabulous friends, a great stable family life, my husband is supportive of my personal freedoms and I don't dwell on negative things or people — they have no place in my life.'

And in a flurry of hugs, laughter and energy, the Queen of Dragons Abreast is off to train for Abreast in Australia 2007 in Caloundra!

Hello dear FOAMs

This will be a very busy 10 days so I thought I'd fill you in!

I will be flat out at work for the next three days with Manager's meetings, filming an Extra story for 9, and a photography day at work, compering a Breakfast celeb debate and then hosting a PR lunch!!!

On Thursday morning I go into RB Hospital to get my port-a-cath (a plastic sleeve inserted into one of the veins of the heart to allow my chemo and any other IVs into my blood system). I have to get this because my veins in my left arm have collapsed and the medicos can't use my right arm (to prevent lymphoedema) for IVs. I get back from surgery for a little rest then get my chemo pumped through the port — a whole lot easier than the last time.

I then have a little 'rest' in hospital until Friday and am thinking 'positive' thoughts about coming home on Friday afternoon!!! I am also being very positive that, with the port, all my bad reactions to chemo will be just a bad nightmare. Kathleen is giving me what she tells me is a 'great hospital read' for the days so I am looking forward to an enforced, but wonderful, rest! And that does NOT include feeling ill!!!

I will have Saturday at home (Ben, Kylie and Madeleine Kate over for dinner whilst we cheer the Wallabies in the Bledisloe

Cup on TV and then Maddie stays the night with Grandfather and 'Gwannie'.) I then go away for our work offsite planning three days.

How lucky am I to have such an interesting time! So will catch up with you next week.

Again, thank you to all of you for your amazing support, love, prayers and friendship. It is what keeps me going each day with a big fat smile!

Smile

AM

Ros Kelly's Journey

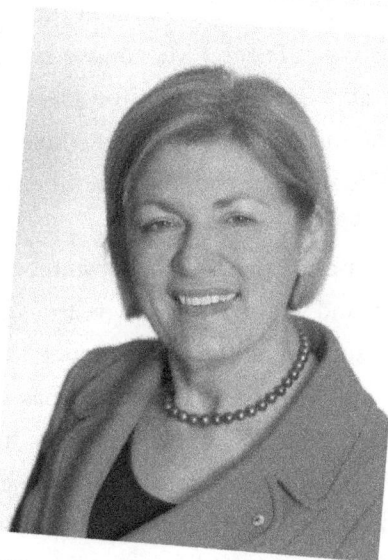

'I didn't want to go public about my cancer because I knew
I couldn't cope with that at this emotional time. I really didn't
want anyone to know. I just wanted to deal with it in my
own little circle.'

os Kelly AO presents as a strong woman, and that's the way she's tried to live her life. 'I like to think of myself as a woman of control, strength and courage. An action woman. If there is something to be done I don't shirk it; I get into action mode and just deal with whatever the problem is.'

But when it came to dealing with her breast cancer diagnosis in 2001, the superwoman was floored and suddenly very vulnerable.

Ros Kelly is a leading female figure in the history of Australian politics. She was a member of the Australian House of Representatives from 1980 to 1995, having spent five years in the ACT Parliament. She was the first Australian Federal MP to give birth while in office and when she was appointed Minister for Defence, Science and Personnel she became the first female Labor Minister, in the House of Representatives. She subsequently held six other portfolios whilst in Parliament.

Nearly 12 months after the so-called 'whiteboard sports rorts affair', Ros left politics and worked for many years as a very successful senior management executive in the environmental arena.

In her political and corporate roles, Ros has always been an extremely busy woman who was in command of her own destiny. But it was the daunting challenge of breast cancer that gave her a new perspective on life and indeed ignited a new passion — something she says that her previous experiences had prepared her for.

'I was certainly an organised woman in charge of my life and just got on and did things. Fitness was always an important part of that life and I never thought for a second that I would be one of the breast cancer statistics. I just didn't fit into any of the "at risk" profiles,' she says.

She had regular mammograms as part of her health consciousness, 'but when I went it was always with the view it was never going to be me. And that was the mental attitude I went with for that critical mammogram, which was just one component of my regular health check-ups. Some calcification showed up and I was referred to a specialist. The doctor wasn't overly concerned and suggested I come back in six months' time. So I didn't give it any further consideration,' she says.

Diligently she returned for the follow-up mammogram to a private radiographer in the suburbs six months later.

'As well as the mammogram, an ultrasound was performed. The woman who was doing the tests recognised me and obviously liked my politics because she spent a lot of time with me. When I'm a little scared, my defence mechanism is to talk a lot and so we chatted about politics, the Labor Party, and just about general women's stuff. I left with the envelope with the films for my doctor never thinking there would be anything sinister about the results.'

Ros was hosting a lunch at her home that day and quickly adopted the hostess role. After the guests left she opened the results envelope and read that the radiographer had noted that there was an area of concern but she says, 'I didn't worry about it at all — that's definitely not me!

'When I went back to the specialist, Dr Crea, he told me I needed a biopsy as he did have some concerns. He reassured me and told me not to worry. I was going to just get on with my life and I still didn't believe for a second that the result was going to be positive.'

At that time Ros was working with one of the world's largest environmental management consultancies, ERM, and on that day she had a meeting with a major electricity company out at Blacktown about environmental training for their top staff.

'I hadn't cancelled anything because I didn't realise how serious my tests were and so I just continued on with my busy life. At this stage I was still certain that the tests would not return a positive result. But having to have a biopsy and then carry on as if nothing else important was happening was more difficult than I expected,' she admits.

'That night I went to see the musical *Shout* with my sister and sister-in-law. I told my sister that I'd had the biopsy that day and the look of horror on her face expressed shock and fear. I remember it was just like a foreboding that this was going to be a disaster for me.

'Next morning I went to the doctor for my results and he walked around the consulting table, took my hand and gently told me the small lump was malignant. I had breast cancer. It was just before Easter and I was horrified. I was in a state of total shock. I couldn't believe it was me. I kept denying the possibility that it could be me because I didn't fit into any profiles. I'd gone from a person who was in control of my life to someone who was absolutely out of control.

'All of a sudden nothing really mattered: jobs, presentations, future plans were no longer relevant. I just wanted to go away to a place I felt safe. So being terribly upset I knew I just needed to be with my husband, David, who was then CEO at Westpac.

'We went to a coffee shop in Martin Place and I was crying; I put my arms around him, sobbing that I had breast cancer. David was also in shock, and we started talking seriously. Strangely, my son, Ben, was walking across Martin Place after school that day and saw us upset and he literally went white. I asked him to sit down with us and I said, "I have something to tell you."

'I looked him straight in the face and told him I had breast cancer. His face lit up and he smiled and said, "Ma, I thought you were going to tell me you and Dad were splitting up. I am so relieved." But then I had to talk to the two of them about fighting this disease as a family.

'Unfortunately, I had gone for all the tests and got my results by myself and so I really didn't remember anything I was told. So now, one of the things I always tell other women is to take someone with them for appointments — so they can listen for you.'

Once Ros had told her family, she was keen to get treatment organised as soon as possible. 'I wanted Dr Crea to operate immediately so that I could take control of my life as soon as possible. But he wanted me to wait until after Easter to give me time to come to terms with the cancer.

'I was still in shock and I was struggling with the fact that the cancer was in my body. I am an action person and it was awful having to wait to do something. But I was helped enormously by the mother of one of my daughter's friends. She had had cancer many years earlier and she turned up one day and said to me, "Ros, the doctors will do fine. They will get this cancer out of your body. What you've got to deal with is your head." And she sat down with me and talked me through how she, as a young mother of two young children, had got through. It made me feel so much better because I thought that if she could do it in a much worse position than I, then surely I could get through it, too. She was a beacon for me on that miserable Easter,' says Ros gratefully.

This was the first time in her life that Ros had had to confront her mortality. So, like most women in her situation, she decided she needed to know as much about the disease as possible.

'I went to lots of websites, and they sent me really nutty. So when that didn't work for me, I trolled the bookshops for books on women living with cancer — but they made me even crazier. The more I read in these dreadful books, the more I kept thinking, "This is really appalling."

'But then my spirits were lifted that holiday period when a friend rang me. She has had a terrible time with breast cancer herself but she was so positive and upbeat that I started to believe I could be okay. She sent me a gift which was very different from the usual gifts of books on living with cancer. She gave me a box of chocolates and a copy of the movie *Chocolat*. It was so uplifting to receive a gift for the future rather than one dealing with death. It pulled me out of survival mode into looking forward to the rest of an exciting life,' Ros says with a smile.

After Easter the lumpectomy was scheduled. 'From that time on, I was fine. My friend had been right: the doctors looked after my body and I was feeling much more optimistic about my life. I didn't look back and I became my old positive self again. I admit I was still a little fragile, but I was a lot stronger than I had been.'

Ros had not told anyone except family and close friends about her diagnosis. 'I didn't want to go public about my cancer because I knew I couldn't cope with that at this emotional time. I really didn't want anyone to know. I just wanted to deal with it in my own little circle.

'But I did make one big mistake. I wanted to protect my children from any publicity and from the worry of my cancer, especially Jess, my daughter, who was doing her HSC. So I tried to do it all by myself,' she confesses. 'My husband was running a bank, so I didn't also want him to have any more pressure. It was a mistake not to let my family support and help me more.

'I had the operation on a Tuesday. Of course I was scared, but I knew I had to have it, so I thought to myself, "Let's just do it; get it over with." From then, I knew I was going to be okay.'

After the operation, Ros was delighted to see that she had both her breasts and a reasonably small scar. She felt no pain and although tired and teary, she was happy for it all to be over.

'I am always a glass half-full girl and I had never found my essence and sense of being depended on the size or shape of my breasts, so my upbeat nature kicked in. I knew I had another journey ahead of me but as I'm not a person who over-analyses, I just got on with it.'

But the timing of her operation could not have been worse considering the stress the family was already under. 'David's half-yearly results for the bank were coming out at the end of the week on Friday morning. I'd come through surgery but the pathology results were due to come through on Friday. The waiting and worrying is hard at any time, but worrying how David could prepare his economic report, especially if the results were bad, was too heavy a burden to carry at the time. So I begged my doctor to get me the results on Thursday night so that David could handle his press conference on Friday morning with less stress. He would have come to grips with whatever my results showed.

'I'd gone home and just waiting for those results to come through on Thursday was the longest day of my life. Finally, around five o'clock in the afternoon, I rang David and asked him to ring my doctor because I just couldn't take that phone call myself. Here was I — a really strong woman — and I just could not make that call. About an hour later David rang and he said he was coming home early and to get the champagne out because the cancer hadn't spread to the nodes and the tumour was low grade. David gave his media conference with no one at all aware of what the family had been through that week.'

Ros did not require chemotherapy and her radiotherapy sessions were to begin at the end of May. 'I went by myself to the treatments. I was still working so I'd go to work each morning, then pop over to the hospital and go home before the kids came home from school. So, from their perspective, once I'd had the operation it was all fixed and over. They were getting on with their lives and as far as they could see I was getting on with mine,' she explains.

'I feel now that I should have included the kids more, especially Jess. I perhaps should have told both children how I was feeling and a lot more about the effect the diagnosis and the treatments had on me. Afterwards, Jess said she'd felt a little excluded, but at the time I thought I was protecting her so she could focus on her HSC. However, on reflection, I think I misjudged her and she probably had the maturity to cope and to support me.

'As I continued going each day I became very conscious of the struggles of many of the other women. I became very close to an older Italian woman who came each day with her daughter. I appreciated how difficult this journey was for many of the women from the country, or those that were not financially well off or those who grappled with young children and those who were alone. But I still wasn't strong enough to do anything about it at that time.

'After about Week 3 of radiation, I had to make a decision. My husband, in his position with Westpac, had to fly to Singapore for an international banking conference. All the top banks were represented and it was a very important meeting. It was one of those conferences where spouses really mattered. So I discussed with my radiographer if I could miss one day to enable me to attend two days in Singapore. He agreed, so I had my radiation early, jumped on a plane for Singapore, attended two dinners, several official functions and hopped back on a plane to Sydney late one night so I could have my next dose of radiation early the next morning.

'Just before I flew out, I sat next to John MacFarlane, the CEO of ANZ Bank, at the dinner. As I started to leave, he grabbed my hand, held it and said, "I am giving you my energy." What an amazing gift from a man who headed a competitor bank to David. And I did carry that energy back with me.'

At that conference Ros also met an amazing woman who changed her outlook on her health crisis. 'Lady Connie Middleton was with her husband from Barclays Bank in London. She'd heard I was in the middle of treatment for breast cancer. One day, walking in the street, she put her arms around me and said, "Don't worry. I had it 20 years ago and just look at me. I'm fine!" I felt an enormous strength from someone who had been on my journey and was okay. It was that spirit of being okay that lifted me up and gave me hope.'

Radiation continued to wear Ros down, and it was around this time she met Margaret Wright, who had only a year earlier finished her own breast cancer journey. 'Margaret gave me some very wise advice. She told me to take a break when I finish radiation because I would recover much faster. I had planned to accompany David on a business trip to London, but I was so tired I suggested Ben go with him and Jess and I would have a quiet week at Port Douglas. For the whole week she studied and I slept. I had to let go of everything. It was incredibly hard for me to let go, but I was forced to acknowledge that breast cancer was changing my life. I had never really recognised the huge physical impact the disease had had on my body. It forced me to concede I was now a different person,' she recalls.

Ros then began her medication. 'I put up with that for five years. It was not a happy combination, me and Tamoxifen!' she grimaces. 'Going five years with the sweats and without a good night's sleep was really difficult. But I had to do it because it is my nature to do the right thing and I was going to do every single thing that protected me from getting a recurrence of the cancer.

'At this time I didn't realise I wasn't one hundred per cent. I just got on with life in what I thought was my usual fashion, trying to be as normal as possible. I had talked with my doctor because I felt I was going crazy and I did take some herbal supplements that helped me a little. But once I stopped taking the drug I became conscious of how I had not been all that well. Finally, after five years of hell, I felt fighting fit again.'

As she is such a well-known public figure, Ros had been very determined to keep her cancer diagnosis under wraps. She had not wanted to be in the public eye when dealing with the disease, nor did she want to add pressure to her family. However, a few months after she finished treatments, the story was leaked to the *Canberra Times*.

'My cancer was now out in the public arena. I wanted to start working to help others but I knew I couldn't take a leadership role in this area until I recovered my own strength. Once I felt I had dealt with my own situation, I was ready to help others. I felt it was very important to give all women — particularly rural women — easy access to information and peer support. So I believed that setting up an information website would be very valuable. It was exciting for me because it was something practical I could do. I knew very little about IT but I'm not bad at marketing. My friend Margaret Wright was an expert in technology so we were a perfect combination to provide this service. This has now been taken over by the National Breast Cancer Centre and has been developed into their official website,' she says proudly.

'So after this website had been launched around Australia I wanted to be more proactive and I was invited to work with the research side. In 2003 I joined the board of the National Breast Cancer Foundation. It became quite clear they wanted me to chair the organisation, although that wasn't in my head at all. I felt I needed some distance between my diagnosis and an active involvement.

'I was still running away from the death cycle and I still felt a little vulnerable. I was struggling with the spectre of people dying from cancer and still experiencing ongoing difficulties with Tamoxifen. I wanted to do my bit, but I wasn't ready to do it full time. But the main reason was I was scared, really scared, I'd have to confront death all the time,' she bravely reveals.

'Eventually, and very reluctantly, I accepted the role of chair. It wasn't that I didn't want to take it on but I was anxious about where it would take me. And I haven't looked back since. It has taken me on the most wonderful journey with fabulous people. There are obviously dark sides when one of our volunteers or speakers or supporters dies.' She pauses. 'Those deaths still really knock me down.

'By and large I am very excited about my role with the NBCF. This is certainly the most stimulating thing I have ever done — looking to find a cure for this dreadful disease. All my previous experiences in politics, business and public life have given me a great platform to be of value in the Foundation. It gives us an entrée to leaders in both the influential public and private sector. I feel we can really create something that is so important for all Australian women.

'There are so many exciting research projects happening every day. Wouldn't it be wonderful if we could get that big breakthrough, like a simple, inexpensive test for breast cancer? Early detection is of the essence so research is the absolute key,' she tells me with contagious enthusiasm.

'The reason I am walking around today is because that one woman doing my tests found the cancer that was tinier than a pinhead — early detection saved me. I could say God was on my side, but I want that for everyone. A world where breast cancer is no longer a death knell would be beautiful.'

As we pack up ready to finish our chat, Ros tells me a story that emphasises for her — as a woman who has had breast cancer — the importance of giving back.

'I was driving back from a weekend away with two young girls who had lost their mother five years ago to breast cancer. The girls were chatting away happily and on that highway it struck me that what I'm doing in the Foundation is protecting these two little girls. We — me and all those other generous women giving back — are not really doing this for ourselves; we are doing it for our daughters and our granddaughters. That's why I do it.'

From: AnneMarie
Subject: BLOODY HELL
Sent: 24 July 2003

Hello dear friends

Just arrived home and thought I'd let you know that I wasn't
able to have chemo today as my blood levels were too low.
My neutrophils were very low. These are the part of the white
blood cells that look after your immune system. To safely
have chemo they need to be at least 1.5%, but mine were
under 0.9%. I asked was it possible to have the chemo today
as I had really psyched myself for it. But alas, the answer was
that if they gave it to me it could kill me. Now I thought that
was a little melodramatic, but my doc assures me she would
NOT risk me!

Funny, as I have felt the healthiest since being diagnosed.
I've been running again and even doing the step runs!
I guess good health and fitness has little to do with
neutrophils. Doc Liz assured me there is absolutely nothing I
can do about my blood levels, so I am not beating myself up
on this.

So I now will have chemo on Tuesday, staying in till Thursday
or Friday. In future I will have my chemo in hospital for
36 hours with an immune booster to ensure I have a
safe level for my immune system. I guess it hasn't really
recovered from the Toxic shock of 2000!

The good news is that I was still able to have my surgery to
insert a port a cath into my chest for chemo delivery (wonder

if I can get a Champagne fill as well???). The op went very
smoothly and although I now have two more scars from
a line of stitches, I will have much easier chemo delivery.
And my blood tests will be less stressful.

I am now looking forward to a great weekend ... and will be
ready on Tuesday!

Smiles and big hugs

AnneMarie

Di Ryall's Journey

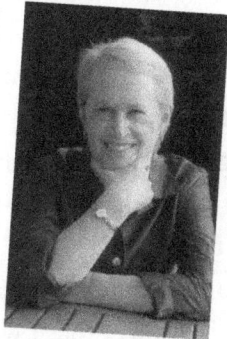

' ... he prescribed diet, meditation, acupuncture and Chinese pills ... I felt extremely confident and comfortable about his advice. I bounced back well from chemo and had hardly any burns from the radiation. I am convinced his different approach really helped me get through more easily.'

As the Managing Director of Apple Australia, Diana Ryall was a busy energetic woman who commanded admiration and respect. She'd been with the company for 18 years and had held the CEO position for four years after literally working her way to the top of the company.

Her days were long, filled with important meetings and decision-making. In October 2000 she was still busy with meetings and decisions, only this time they concerned not the growth and development of a huge corporation but the continuation of her own life.

After being diagnosed with breast cancer in 2000, Di maintained her Chief Executive position with Apple, but could only work in a part-time capacity during her treatment.

'My prognosis wasn't great, so I decided that I must do everything I could to stay alive. I also set myself a goal of reducing the likelihood of the cancer returning in two years.

'Life at Apple was relentless and demanding. I decided at the end of my medical treatments for cancer that I would either need to get fully back into the high-stress job of CEO again or take the decision to step down. I also knew that, at that time, my overwhelming first priority was to remove all significant stress in my life. So I stepped down from my job at the end of 2001. I knew that people would understand.

'Too often, managers stay on longer than they should. I always knew I wasn't going to stay in the position for ever, and this seemed like the right time for me — especially as I felt that others would appreciate that my concerns for my health and wellbeing came first,' Di says.

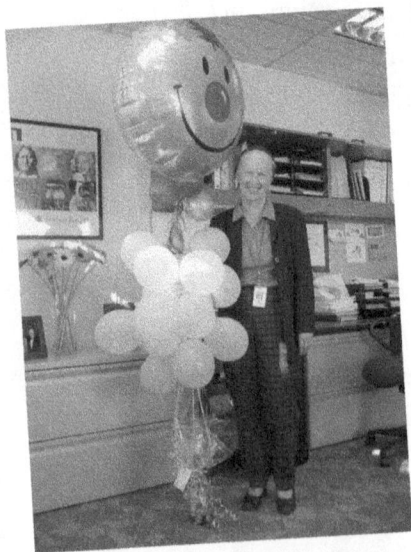

Support from Di's corporate colleagues

'Once it was confirmed that I had breast cancer, I was very open about my diagnosis. I sent a group email to everyone at Apple so that they all knew. That gave the staff permission to be open and frank and also, by being candid, people were prepared to talk to me about the disease. A media release was sent out so my diagnosis was out in the public arena. Everyone was very supportive,' she adds.

Di and I meet in a quaint coffee shop to talk about her journey. Casually dressed and very relaxed, she explains that it was a hard decision to make — but the right one.

'I know I made the best decision for me. All the medical fraternity acknowledge that lack of exercise and excess weight are not conducive to good health and when I was working long hours at Apple, those factors were difficult to control. What researchers haven't yet identified is what impact stress does have on our bodies. I have no doubt my decision to forego corporate life for a healthier, less stressful existence is the reason we are here chatting today.'

After her treatment, Di was very focused on doing everything in her power to survive the next two years cancer-free and then to keep living every year after that, one at a time. As a high-level executive, Di was used to setting goals and being focused on achieving milestones. She was also going to use — and need — every bit of her professional acumen in her approach to beating cancer.

'One of the things that shattered me with my diagnosis was that I might not see my grandchildren, let alone be there when they were growing up. But I have realised that goal with the birth of my little granddaughter and more recently my first grandson, so that is a blessing. I have also reached 60 and that was another important landmark for me. Now I am determined to keep setting these markers for the future.

'Before I was diagnosed I knew quite a bit about breast cancer as my best friend, Margie, died of the disease at only 37. It was tragic; she died within months of her diagnosis, leaving two small children. However, I didn't know much about the disease medically and I actually saw it as a death sentence,' says Di.

'I don't know how other people react, but when I was diagnosed it was an incredible shock. My grandmother had lived to the ripe old age of 101, and since I was only 53, I figured I was about halfway through my life. But with the diagnosis, I realised that my life was already precarious and would be significantly changed. That was certainly something I had difficulty in facing.'

Di explains that although there was no family history of breast cancer, both she and her mother had very lumpy breasts, and Di had had a benign lump removed when she was 30. 'It was innocent, just a cyst, but it made me vigilant.

'I had taken two weeks' leave in 2000 to enjoy the Sydney Olympics here in my home city. Earlier in the year, Apple received the Hewitt Associates Australian Employer of the Year Award, which gave me great pride as the Australian leader. Life was exciting and I thought nothing of going off for my annual breast check-up and mammogram.

'I had absolutely no inkling that anything was wrong, although in hindsight I suppose I should have guessed something was just not quite right. One of my nipples was slightly out of alignment, but I knew I had put on some weight and I discarded the notion that there was a problem as ridiculous. I thought I just needed to go out and buy new, correctly fitted bras.'

'My lump was directly behind the nipple and could not be felt easily, and my skin hadn't changed. It never occurred to me that there was anything wrong, and certainly not anything sinister. When I walked into the doctor's surgery I didn't expect there would be anything significantly the matter with me. But suddenly I had two doctors in the room asking me about the nipple slant. They suggested they do a biopsy and told me right upfront they were 90 per cent sure I had breast cancer.' A tremor in Di's voice betrays the emotion brought on by that blunt assessment.

The doctors were also worried about several other unusual lumps in Di's breast that had been revealed by her mammogram and ultrasound. Di received her biopsy results from her GP the next day.

'It was a Friday, late in October 2000. I don't know exactly what date because I decided that was one date I wasn't going to enter in my memory,' says Di.

'The instant I walked in to my doctor, I knew it was bad news. She had put my appointment fairly late in the day to ensure she had the results and that she could make time to talk with me. She was really good. After delivering the bad news, she reminded me that cancer isn't always a death sentence. But when you get this sort of news, you really don't listen. You are in so much emotional pain and disbelief that it is really hard to take in positive messages,' Di says perceptively.

'I'm glad I took my husband, Bill, to the appointment because I really don't remember too much of what was said. One minute my life was looking good; now I was devastated that everything was about to change. I had done all my check-ups, took good care of myself and I never thought it would be me. I wasn't naïve but I did have the view that once you are diagnosed with cancer there was very little chance of long-term survival.

'It's funny, isn't it?' she says. 'When people are given the bad news and they say, "Well, I just got on with it," you wonder if they really did, or were they terrified and just said that? I don't think we can ever underestimate the impact of bad news.

'On the day I had the mammogram — before the diagnosis — I rang my PA and told her that things weren't looking too good and I wasn't really up to coming in and asked her to cancel all my appointments for that day.

'I'm pretty tough and resilient, but I was so shaken at the clinic with the suggestion that I could possibly have breast cancer that I knew I couldn't drive myself home. I called Bill, who collected me and took me home. It's a running joke in the family that when things get tough we sit down and have a cup of tea — so that's all I could do. Sit down with a cuppa.'

Di had to then make decisions about how to tell her family and friends. She and Bill had planned a dinner party for friends the

Saturday following her diagnosis; they made a decision to go ahead with the party but to not tell anyone.

However, the day after the party she rang each of the guests and broke the news to them. 'It caused a bit of a hooha, and they were disappointed not to have known, but I really wanted to just enjoy myself and forget — even if it was only for that one night.'

'I phoned my sons straight away, and although I don't want to recall that day, my son Peter, who was in Townsville with the army, remembers the call. Sadly, he had been away when our close family friend died, and he was also overseas when his grandmother died. So it wasn't nice to deliver bad news to him via the phone once again.

'My other son, Scott, was in town and came straight over. Ironically, his girlfriend's mother had been diagnosed nine months earlier with breast cancer, so he understood.'

Di's gut reaction to her diagnosis was shock and, understandably, she wasn't happy about it, 'but in these type of situations I don't do the anger or bargaining with God. Instead, I go straight into information-gathering mode. So I immediately hit the book stores and bought several books. One of them was called *Your Life in Your Hands*, and when I showed Bill, he told me he knew the author, Jane Plant. She was a geochemist and so when she was diagnosed with breast cancer and had five reoccurrences — everyone thought she was going to die — she turned to research in her quest to live. Although she covered a lot of other ground, she was particularly interested in diet and its role in controlling our health.

'When I opened the front cover, I saw that the acknowledgments mentioned the husband of my friend Margie, who had died. I am a believer in serendipity and when I looked at that I absolutely knew I was meant to read this book,' she says. 'It had a series of diet suggestions that I implemented immediately.'

Although she believed she had always eaten in a healthy way, Di changed her diet the day after she was diagnosed. She cut out all dairy — a choice she has stuck to — 'because research into diets shows that Chinese and Japanese women, who eat fish, use soy products and rice, have very little incidence of breast cancer,' Di explains. She also cut out red meat and increased her daily consumption of vegetables.

'So I really made major changes to my diet and it all started with that book. Intriguing things happened. The book explains that the Chinese think we Westerners smell of sour milk. Amazingly, soon after I gave up dairy foods I noticed that I didn't need a deodorant any more. Previously it was a problem, and I was always looking for stronger deodorant brands, but not any more. I will always believe that cutting dairy out of my diet had a hugely positive impact on my body.'

Di laughingly says I can think she is 'a raving looney' but she is quite certain that after switching to soy, she could feel things changing in her breast in the first week. 'It was like my breast was clearing itself out, getting rid of impurities. I still find it intriguing that when I had the mastectomy 17 days after changing my diet, there were three spots in the breast and the doctors were absolutely stunned: they were very low-grade. Given that there had been nothing in the breast tissue 12 months earlier, the tumour had to be fast-growing. The doctors were very surprised, but I wasn't. I put it down totally to the fact I changed my diet radically. I am sure it wasn't psychosomatic; it was like my breast was releasing all the toxins in there,' Di says assuredly.

As normally happens, Di went quickly on what she calls a 'surgeon hunt'. I called everyone who I thought could help me find the best doctor for me.' She made two appointments, both of whom were recommended to her as excellent surgeons.

'The first man was a delightful person but I felt like I was really a specimen. He went through everything he thought I should know but in what I suspect is the natural style for surgeons. I needed information, but I also needed to be involved as a person — someone who was in a challenging situation.

'The second doctor, whom I selected, treated me holistically — as a whole person who had a problem. Importantly for me, she recognised that only part of my predicament was medical and much of it was emotional. We talked through all the options and I decided to go with her.'

Di didn't want to rush into her surgery and so took a holiday weekend with her girlfriends. 'They all knew what was happening, but before I was on the medical treadmill it was just nice to stop and enjoy life and friendships. I also think too many women feel they have to rush immediately into surgery. I didn't think a week or two would make a difference medically and this gap time allowed my brain to get around the diagnosis.'

When Di had her mastectomy she wasn't really upset about how the loss of a breast would look physically, 'it was more a sadness that my breasts had served me well feeding my boys. Losing the breast felt like giving up a part of me and part of my history.'

Several days after the operation Di was told there was cancer in seven of her lymph nodes. She then needed to work out with her multidisciplinary team what treatment regime would be best for her.

'With my oncologist, I talked through all the options presented to me and considered their impact on my longevity. I accepted the team's advice to submit myself to the full course of therapies — two rounds of chemotherapy, radiation therapy and a five-year course of medication. However, I still really struggled with the fact that two weeks ago I felt I was perfectly healthy and here I was discussing survival rates.'

Di admits the most difficult thing for her to cope with at this time was the emotional effects her unexpected diagnosis was having on her. Being a self-confessed numbers person, she really struggled to see a 75 per cent survival rate as good news. 'In any other situation, you'd reckon that was great odds, but I must admit my mind kept putting me down into the bottom 25 per cent.

'Having accepted that I was going to have to go through chemotherapy was daunting, but there was light from the gloom for me when my oncologist asked if I drank alcohol. On hearing that I liked a drink or two, she'd told me that was good news because my liver was used to dealing with chemicals,' she laughs.

'So I faced the full-on chemical attack with four treatments of "red devil" chemo, followed by radiation therapy, with another four chemo sessions of Taxol. I must admit it is very confronting seeing the staff dressed in what looks like full combat gear come in and pump the chemicals through my body. I'd read about people imagining soldiers going into war against the cancer, but it didn't reduce my hesitation.'

Women react as individuals during their treatments. Some check out of personal responsibility, handing over their lives to the medical staff; others want information but only enough to participate in decision-making. Di admits that she 'spent way too much time on the web researching and reading lots and lots of different views and opinions — gathering all the knowledge and data I could.

'During that time I met a friend of a friend for coffee. It was the first time that I actually sat down with someone else and talked openly about how I felt to have my life threatened. The woman had three little girls under the age of five and had the extremely rare, but most often terminal, placental cancer. She had found a Chinese doctor who had both Eastern and Western qualifications and she felt was helping her survive.

'This was exciting news for me. I went and saw the doctor and he prescribed diet, meditation, acupuncture and Chinese pills. On his advice, I went off all the Chinese medicine for about a week around chemo. I felt extremely confident and comfortable about his advice. I bounced back well from chemo and had hardly any burns from the radiation. I am convinced his different approach really helped me get through more easily,' says Di confidently.

'He made me feel so determined and positive about building up my T-cells and my general health that I have continued to see him for the past five years. During that time I was taking Tamoxifen, so I was very happy to combine Western and Eastern medicine. In fact, I would do anything that would ensure I could achieve my goal of surviving for the first two years without a reoccurence.'

He was also very strict about my diet, which also focused on consuming no dairy, no red meat, only organic chicken and lots of fruit and vegetables. The treatment was a significant financial outlay, because you get nothing back from medical insurance, but I saw it as an invaluable investment in my future good health.'

Di is also pleased that alternative methods of treating breast cancer are now being looked into and their effects analysed in a number of research programs.

'When I look back now, I wonder if my diet in the years preceding my diagnosis was actually the cause of my breast cancer — too much dairy and to compensate for the stress of my job I had taken to eating lots of sweets?' Di asks.

Di attributes her choices in medicines and diet as being responsible for her recovery, and indeed survival. However, it was on a psychological level that she continued to struggle. After she finished chemotherapy she went to a psychologist because 'I still had trouble coming to grips with what this meant for my life,' she says honestly. 'I wasn't ready to check out of living and he was really helpful in allowing me to see a future.

'One of the things he asked me to do was to stand on the far end of a carpet facing out and visualise the end of my life. In a moment of clarity I realised my life wasn't over. We never know how much of our life is yet to be lived, but that whatever time is left must be enjoyed and savoured. Every day is important.'

Di agrees with many survivors of breast cancer that the most challenging period during a woman's journey with breast cancer is the time following the end of medical treatments. 'Whilst you are busy with all the medical appointments, you survive and are propelled forwards by the next treatment. Then all of a sudden you are finished and the medical carers wave goodbye and tell you they'll see you in six months' time. I tried hard to be positive about surviving, but it is scary being on your own. Every pain or ache seems to spell doom.'

Di confesses that it took her ages to use the past tense about cancer and she is still inclined to say that she was diagnosed *with* breast cancer in 2000, rather than in 2008, be definitive about having *had* cancer. It is a subtle difference in words, but quite an important distinction in meaning.

'In the past I had a lot of urgency in my life. I was due to travel overseas with friends in the May of 2001, during the time when I was having treatment, but they were happy to postpone the trip and go later in that year in October. We did go away but as I wasn't that long over treatments I was still a little slow on my feet. Such a simple thing forced me to be less earnest and more relaxed,' she adds thoughtfully.

'So whilst I have lost the stressfulness of having to continually achieve and get things done, I do still have an urgency. But now it is to do as much as I can with my life — because who knows what is in the future. Now I do everything sooner rather than later. I don't want to have regrets, so if I wish for something, then I do it now. I did write down the 100 things I want to experience before I die, and I probably need to revisit that. But the interesting thing now is that I am much more comfortable with myself and the life I am living.

'In fact, there aren't that many things I want to do before I die,' she says. 'I do want to be around for my grandchildren, but materialism isn't anywhere as high on the list as it used to be. I am pretty well roosting in my community and certainly much more protective of my body and my mind now.'

Di says breast cancer gave her the opportunity to take stock of life, face her demons and place value on different things now. She appreciates being well, being healthy and not having to visit doctors all the time. She nurtures those who matter to her.

Facing the future with optimism is Di's key to getting on with her new life. She feels comfortable that she has done everything she could have done to live a long life. If the cancer comes back, she says she will give it her best shot.

'We all know people who have the cancer come back, so I am keeping myself in the best possible condition to endure. If I have to fight again I am prepared to do so.'

When Di resigned from Apple in 2001, she decided not to go back to the big top end of business. 'I didn't want to be in corporate life in the same full-on way I had been. So I guess I just hung around until 2002 when I started to look for inspiration.

'I had noticed in speaking to young women that they felt corporate life was often very difficult. So in August 2002 I tentatively started a mentoring style business for young women. It immediately took off, with 24 young businesswomen signing up for a six-month program. The business expanded and now my company, Xplore for Success, is partnering with many of the major organisations in Australia and I have a team of fabulous women working with me. We stimulate, teach, inspire and motivate young women who aspire to build their career,' Di says proudly.

Professionally and personally, Di is confident and flying high. However, on a personal level, her fear of mortality, of facing her own death, still hovers around her. 'I do struggle with the question of what happens if I die and who is going to look after the business and the programs. Because we never know when it is our time, that is one thing I continue to grapple with so I guess that prompts me to get a move on and do my succession plan,' admits Di. 'But working in an area that is making a difference in the world through the mentoring programs, gives me energy and great satisfaction.'

It is her faith in alternative treatments that gives her the courage to face the future boldly. By taking control of what she does, how she thinks, what she eats and contributing to a better world, Di feels that she is finally in a comfortable place in her life.

From: AnneMarie
Subject: ITCHY MAN SYNDROME
Sent: 30 July 2003

Lovely FOAM friends

Well, chemo 3 has finally happened! Lucky my current theme is *always look on the bright side of life* because I am being given lots of opportunities to do so! But each is a new challenge to face and achieve and another wonderful life growth experience.

I certainly have learned the meaning of *In God's time, not AnneMarie's*.

After having the chemo delayed from Thursday last week, I was psyched up and very relaxed, knowing that the port would make the chemo flow in easily with little stress to my body. But sometimes life is a comedy acted out!

I arrived at 11.30am after leaving my work off-site bonding sessions so I could have this thing done. After waiting for a while I went in as they prepared the port site. They then remembered that on Thursday my neutrophils had been very low, so they had to give me a new set of blood tests. Fair enough! By this time, it is about 1pm and fortunately the lunch lady still had a plate of sandwiches and an orange juice left. See: good things do happen!

About 2pm my doctor comes over and tells me that, unfortunately, AGAIN I can't have chemo because I am still neutropenic. And she tells me she is 'a little concerned that in the past 5 days they have remained at exactly the low level of Thursday'.

Jokingly, I asked her did she get the wrong printout? She laughed and said, 'Hey I better check that.' Sheepishly, she comes back saying my new results aren't in yet. Now all my worries about chemo have flown away and my concern is if I am who I am and are they giving me MY treatment. Mental note: check that each time it has my name on it!

By 2.20pm she's back with the right results and the blood is fine and I'm ready to go. So off they go to make up my concoction! Luckily, I have a great hospital book, *Mad About the Boys*, so I am now happily reading away when chief nurse comes up and pulls the curtains around — a sure sign that all is not well in Oncology Land!

'Unfortunately, we have had two seriously ill cases come into the oncology wards and so they've had to take your bed.'

'Fine. I'll just have another one ... I'm easy to please.'

'Well, that's the problem, there are no other beds, and we have another patient in Emergency to get a bed for as well.'

Hmmm, so what do they suggest?

Their suggestion is to postpone my chemo until tomorrow or maybe Thursday. You can imagine how well this went down with me. Whilst maintaining my nice manners (and understanding that in the big picture of ill people I was not near the top), I said I was here and would have chemo today and what other thoughts had she?

Nothing!!!

So I decided that I'd do the chemo and wait for a few hours in the Day Patients area. If I became ill, then they would have to either find a bed in the hospital or at worst send me via Emergency to a ward. If, on the positive side, I felt ok and had kept everything inside me, I would go home. My doctor did offer to do the chemo then ambulance me across to another hospital for the night.

Pete said he would come back from Boonah and delay his flight to Cairns on Wednesday morning. So at least I knew I had someone there in case of problems.

Finally they started the chemo at 3.30pm and finished at 5.15pm. I then discovered the Day Patients closed at 6pm not 8pm as I'd been told. My doctor saw me again and whilst I felt ok then, I knew it took about 1½–2 hours to churn up. Short of sitting in there and making Nurse Ursula miss her netball match, I had to go home. Doc gave me every legal anti-nausea medication she could, so I just figured I'd deal with it as best as I could — with happiness and courage sitting on each shoulder watching over my stomach!

I ordered a cab, and being positive, a beautiful Gold Class one arrived with a charming driver. So sometimes things aren't as bad as they could be ... and again looking on the bright side!

Good news is although I felt very ordinary, enough to sleep with a bucket beside my bed, I woke up tender but whole. The sun shone warmly and a pamper parcel arrived as a surprise from darling daughter Vanesa. So life is always beautiful. And being able to write to you lovely friends makes the yukky bits fade quicker.

I did mean to tell you that during the port op, a funny thing did happen to me and the staff (love them for laughing so much ... NOT) still talk about it. I had to have Vancomycin — an antibiotic — before the operation. The staff forgot to tell me that there are a couple of side effects, even though they don't happen often. But of course I am on a journey of new experiences so, pick me, pick me!

After the drug had been dripped into me for about 30 minutes, I started to feel an itch in my head. Had a bit of a gentle scratch — don't want to knock out the remaining hairs — and then to distract myself went for a walk. I looked in a mirror on the toilet wall and noticed a bright (as in beetroot colour) stripe along my forehead. On leaving the loo, it had descended to my eyebrows. Alerted that this was not my normal colouring, I rang for the nurse, who — bless her little bobby sox (NOT) — laughed at the sight of me tearing into my itchy head with a bright red face. 'OOH,' she said, 'you've got red face itchy man syndrome!' Hell, I didn't care what it was called — just fix it.

So for the next hour I sat with a really cold towel perched in a pirouette style on my head, dripping iced water all over me, hands scrubbing all my hair off to ease the itch and a post-box coloured face. Very attractive. It did eventually go, but the entertainment value for the staff could have been a problem, except I could not stop laughing myself, meaning there was a ward full of jocularity that even had all the other patients laughing. Mind you, my dignified air that I try so hard to conjure up, has lost all credibility. Robin Williams as Doctor Patch had nothing on my clown doctor tactics that day.

So the wonderful saga continues for me. I now only have three more chemos. And yes, I do have hair, although it is a very spunky short and spiky affair that artistically lets you view my scalp from several angles. Doc still marvels at my nearly 7 week survival.

Philosophically, I have learned that physically I have a tough exterior, with my hair etc, but am more vulnerable on the inside, with harsh reactions to drugs and treatments (why didn't I believe in Panadol and pain relief in my past???). I now realise that I can still be strong and keep running and exercising and working full-time, yet I know I need to be quite gentle with my insides.

Maybe on a deeper level this chemical journey has told me some deeper truths about my life and living in general. No matter how tough we try to be on the outside, our true soul is often in need of more love and nurture than we think. So, friends, remember the inner soul and be gentle with it.

Love you all

AM

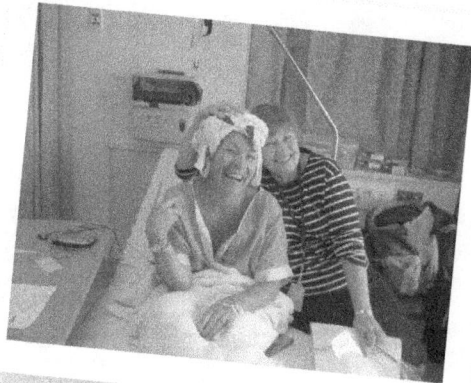

Beverley and Barry Wilson
Share David's Journey

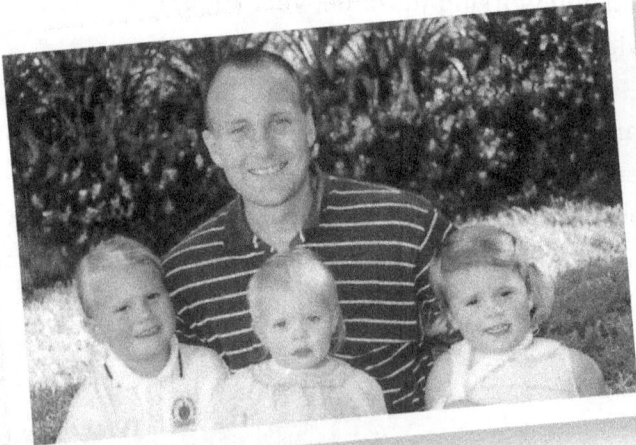

'Through a work colleague of Barry's, we knew that breast cancer could occur in males, but that it was mainly in older men. Because of my dreadful suspicion, and I guess my family experience with my mother's death from breast cancer, I urged David to see somebody.'

When I was diagnosed with cancer I know my children — my son and my daughter — struggled with my journey, unable to do anything but be there for me.

I don't know how I could have coped had the tables been reversed and I'd watched my own child die. Barry and Beverley Wilson lost their son, David, when he was just 32 years old. It is not the natural order of things that parents bury their children. Nor did it seem possible that a fit young man should die of what is widely seen as a woman's disease. However, from my research, I know that 95 new diagnoses of breast cancer are expected in men in Australia each year.

'We lost our son. But life does go on, however difficult at times, but it is never quite the same,' says Beverley.

Father Barry adds, 'It is nine years since David's parting and in some ways it only seems a short while ago, while at the same time it seems a lifetime ago. Strange how one can have such opposing thoughts at the same time.'

'Cancer was a potential enemy lying in wait for the Wilson family,' says Beverley. 'My journey with cancer began over 70 years ago when my maternal grandfather died. Through my childhood I was aware that he had died of cancer, but in all innocence I never believed it was of any great consequence to me.

'Then years later, in 1965, when my mother was 55, she developed breast cancer. Although treatment and knowledge had advanced — for we know doctors used radiotherapy back then — there was obviously a huge amount we did not know. Sadly, four years later, when she was just 60, she passed away. That was in 1969. On her birthday that year we could put a man on the moon, but we could not beat cancer — amazing!' says Beverley.

At that time Beverley and Barry had one son, David, and in the next six years two daughters were added to their family.

Beverley and Barry's pride in their family shines in their faces as they speak. 'We were charmed,' Beverley tells me. 'We had a lovely home, three good healthy children, and life was wonderful. The children

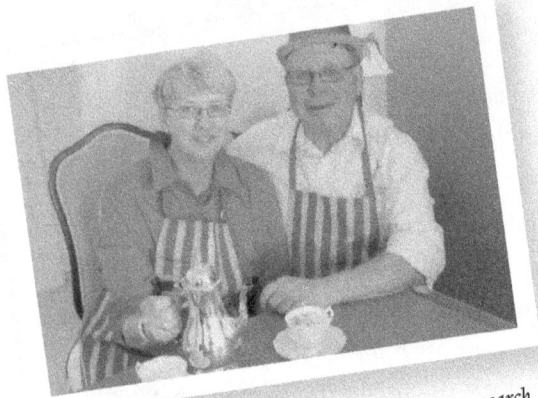

Beverley and Barry fundraising for breast cancer research

all did well at school and played good levels of sport, particularly David.'

'David was a very keen sportsman,' says Barry; he thoroughly enjoyed supporting his son's involvement in sport. 'I have a flood of memories. David and I shared countless hours on the sporting fields. It was a pleasure to get David to school for early-morning training, even though it meant I had to cover many extra miles to go to work. His effort and commitment to cricket and rugby could not have been higher and he really earned his First Cap for cricket as well as the First Rugby Jersey — wearing both with pride.'

Barry also looks back fondly on the family holidays in the snowfields. 'We were all bitten with the snow sports bug. For many years, as a family, we went down to the snowfields three times a year. David and I sometimes went alone — just so we wouldn't forget how to ski.' Barry laughingly adds, 'I had wanted to ski as well as David did but in the end I was content to just be there, not go onto the black runs, and wait to meet him at the bottom.'

By the age of 21 David had graduated from university with Honours in Economics. This led to a job with Credit Suisse in the new Financial Derivatives division, and a year later he was running the Australian book from Tokyo. 'He progressed to running the Yen book, which was the largest in the bank — not, of course, without the stress,' notes Beverley.

In 1994, when he was 26, David returned to Sydney to marry his sweetheart, Emma, the true love of his life. Ten days later, on his return from their honeymoon, David confessed to his mother that he'd found a strange lump in his chest area.

'He didn't know what to do,' says Beverley. 'That afternoon he saw our GP, who I feel was suspicious about the growth, and so the doctor gave David a letter to a surgeon. But as he and Emma were booked on that Friday night plane to Tokyo and he had been away three weeks, he felt he could not stay in Australia any longer. So with incredibly heavy hearts we put them on the plane to begin their new life together in Tokyo.

'Through a work colleague of Barry's, we knew that breast cancer could occur in males, but that it was mainly in older men. Because of my dreadful suspicion — and I guess considering my family experience with my mother's death from breast cancer — I urged David to see somebody in Tokyo. This he did.'

Beverley recalls that the doctor in Japan was puzzled, but presumed it was some sort of female hormone abnormality. 'That diagnosis seemed to satisfy David. But I felt sick with worry and I was very concerned, so I suggested he seek further advice. A week later he did. This second doctor likewise was unsure of the cause of the lump. He suggested he'd measure it and then in six months' time they could measure it again and check if there was any change in the size and appearance of the lump.

'But without sounding like a panic-stricken mother thousands of miles away, I was still very worried. I suggested David seek a biopsy, which fortunately he did. To the doctor's absolute amazement, the lump proved to be malignant. He could not believe the result so he returned it for another examination. It was all too unbelievable for the lump to be cancerous. But when the second set of results came back ten days later, the findings of cancer were the same. And of course our lives were changed for ever,' Beverley says.

Barry will never forget that Monday morning phone call from Tokyo. 'David called me at my office to break the news that the biopsy was malignant and that he had been diagnosed with breast cancer. I was distraught. I had to ring Beverley and I didn't know how I was going to break the news to her,' he confesses. 'How we wished it not to be true.'

When David knew that he was dealing with a potentially fatal disease, he decided to return to Australia for treatment. Barry and Beverley contacted a Sydney surgeon who would operate on him.

'I remember the surgeon stressed that I should tell David to bring the slides of the tissue samples when he returned to Australia. That doctor also struggled to believe David had breast cancer,' says Beverley.

Sadly, the reality was David did have breast cancer. So just six weeks after his wedding, David had a mastectomy. He also had a large number of lymph glands removed, many of which were also cancerous. This now meant chemotherapy and the potential destruction of his fertility.

'This was gut-wrenchingly bad news for everybody,' admits Barry. 'David wanted a family. I was so proud of my son that in the midst of this medical nightmare he remained thoughtful and strong. He delayed the commencement of his chemo treatment for two weeks so that he could visit the sperm bank and put aside sperm for the future.'

Miraculously, Emma conceived naturally and for the next six months David and Emma remained in Sydney. 'It was a time of mixed emotions for all of us,' says Beverley. 'David was coping with his invasive chemo treatments, and Emma was dealing with supporting David as well as her pregnancy.'

In May 1995, 13 months after their wedding, their first daughter was born and David and Emma were happy. Life for the young couple was again rosy so they returned to Tokyo. They knew that for David to recover fully would mean travelling a long, hard road, but they were determined to live a full and contented family life back in Japan.

David researched the disease and learned as much as he could about cancer. He also took a tremendous amount of care and control of his treatment, diet and lifestyle. The couple made many lifestyle changes to ensure David's health improved and then remained good.

Beverley, the devoted grandmother, proudly tells me that 'nine months later, the young couple thought they'd get on with family business. Emma was planning to come to Sydney for insemination, but to their and everyone's amazement, she discovered she had conceived naturally. So in December 1996, their second little daughter was born. You can imagine the delight was sublime with this second miracle,' says Beverley with a smile.

However, this joy only lasted for six months. In the middle of the next year, 1997, and two years after his diagnosis, David realised metastasis had developed.

'It was just before his sister's wedding,' explains Barry. 'We had hoped he was in remission, but sadly this was not so. We were devastated to learn the cancer was back and that now his lungs, ribs, sternum and knee had been affected. Words cannot explain our grief.

'I can tell you, Beverley and I and our whole family were very relieved when David and Emma decided that living in Tokyo was now not possible, and in December 1997 they decided to return to Sydney for further treatment. David's employers, Credit Suisse, continued to totally support David even after their return. They really were a thoughtful, caring and generous employer,' says Barry gratefully.

In the jaws of despair concerning David's secondary cancer, Beverley and Barry again found joy when David announced that a new baby was on the way. 'Miracle of miracles was how we saw Emma's pregnancy,' says Beverley, 'and David's beautiful third daughter was born in August 1998.'

Throughout all this time David was researching treatments around the world, and at one stage made contact with a leading research doctor in Boston, whom he visited. 'The doctor felt there was little more he could recommend for David as the treatment being undertaken in Sydney was as good as anywhere in the world at that time. This was reassuring and a credit to our doctors and clinics,' says Beverley.

David's father, Barry, adds, 'Knowing our son had limited time was very challenging for everyone. We were relieved David stayed in Sydney and stopped working. He used to say, "I am a 30-year-old in a 60-year-old body." It was a difficult time for our family, but it was a blessing to be able to spend this final time with David. Although he wasn't so well, it was lovely being with David's family often and seeing them grow and develop. We also enjoyed that extra time he shared with us, especially those regular Tuesday lunches — just great memories.

'How we hoped and wished those last chemo treatments would work, even if it only gave him another six months or so. But that was not to be. How hard it hit us. I vividly remember that last weekend he was with us — as if he knew the end was close,' Barry says emotionally.

'I remember how he directed very close friends and family to come in as he really wanted to say special things to each of them. It was wonderful how David arranged to have a video taken of him, leaving messages for his three little girls. They will always have that video and their father's messages to them. And through this recording they will know and understand their father's love for them just a little more,' says Barry.

Sadly, in August 2000 when David was 32, he lost his battle with breast cancer just before the Olympics which he so desperately had hoped to see. 'At the end, David's mind became hazy and by the Tuesday evening, his short but full life with us ceased. Yes, we wept and wept and we still do, but I'm forever grateful that he was our son — and indeed that he continues to be,' says Barry with pride.

Beverley takes up the story, adding, 'We'd been on an incredible journey with David — both before his illness and throughout the tough times. I am grateful that we did have longer than the medical fraternity thought. Years later, the original surgeon shared with our eldest daughter, who is a nurse, that at the time of surgery he probably only gave David six months of life. But in fact he survived six years with the help of treatment and lifestyle changes.

'We never expected this tragedy to happen to us. I guess if I have one message to leave with everybody — young and old, male and female — it is to get to know their own body intimately. Recognise any change or abnormality and don't be afraid or hesitate to respond to it. Better to be sure than sorry.'

Following David's death, at Beverley's suggestion, a memorial bench was built and placed at David's alma mater, Newington College.

'Creating the bench was such a lovely idea, and we have found it to be a blessing for us as well as for David's sisters and his wife and children. On his birth and death anniversaries, we spend time at Newington and sit on the bench, which is right behind the goalpost of the Johnson. When possible, our granddaughters come with us,' says Barry.

'David's great school friend, Stu, had been delighted to be asked to make the seat and what a tremendous job he did. Stu had thought of the normal design but decided to build one that encompassed David's many years in Japan, so the back is shaped like the rays of the sun. He told us that it also played on the word sun as David was our "son". It is made from Australian hardwood — just another example of Stu's quiet and thoughtful nature. It stands as a physical testament to David's life and is a quiet focus for all of the family — we can go there, sit, and remember the good times with David.'

Together Barry and Beverley finish telling me David's story saying, 'We don't understand why David's life on this earth was so relatively short, but we do know that those 32 years we did share were some of the most joyous in our journey. Although David is no longer here, we are privileged to love, share and support Emma and their three girls.

'He lost his fight against breast cancer at such a young age. He had so much to look forward to, with a loving wife and three beautiful children, who I consider were just amazing miracles given the circumstances. Our belief in God does not preclude us from the ups and downs of life but it does give us strength and hopefully some peace when turmoil comes calling.

'I have no doubt that David is aware of all this, just as I know his spirit and presence is constantly around us, even though we cannot physically see or touch him.'

From: AnneMarie
Subject: BALD DAY
Sent: 6 August 2003

Well, the day is about to dawn — my B Day. But not that one where I get presents and cake back on April 1st.

No, this is BALD Day.

On Saturday I will wake up with my sparklingly attractive 134 hairs on my head and by lunchtime I will have a shiny pate! That is assuming Ross Coco wields his shears cleanly. And I've borrowed one of granddaughter Madeleine Kate's special 'bald baby head elastics' to make sure I am very fetching!

Saturday is *Bluey Day* — the day around Australia when some brave police and emergency services personnel shave their heads to raise money for children's cancer research. To demonstrate my support for *Bluey Day* I have agreed to have my head shaved — and on TV!

I suddenly realised that this is it! This is the moment of courage for me when baring my head also means baring my soul and baring my identity as a person. I have to admit to a few tears and a real fear. Not only because finally the day of complete hair loss is here, but more because it had finally sunk in that I actually HAD a serious illness. Cancer becomes very real for me. By positively looking ahead every day and never even questioning the fact that I won't be that disgraceful old 94-year-old, I needed this to jolt me into acknowledging how serious my situation was. I'm not dwelling on it, but sometimes I need that message to realise how very blessed I am.

And blessed I am!! I realise what a gift I have been given.
I get to know I can be accepted and loved as me. I am
empowered to be the very best person I can be and not be
encumbered with my physical appearance — God knows,
a bald, middle-aged woman with bad skin, mouth ulcers,
stitched up boob and chest wall and a saggy tummy is hardly
a page 3 girl!!!! And yet I am loved.

I have a chance to be me and, as scary as that is, I am looking
forward to it. (Mind you, ask me how I feel about 6.30pm
Saturday or on Monday morning heading off to work for the
photo shoot I'm doing, hoping it's not too cold! ... the answer
may be more tears.)

So if you're walking down the street and spot a beautifully
bald woman, it just could be me — and if not, she must be
gorgeous too!!

Smiles

AM

PS Important Question: How far do I put my foundation on
with no hairline?

Liddy Clark's Journey

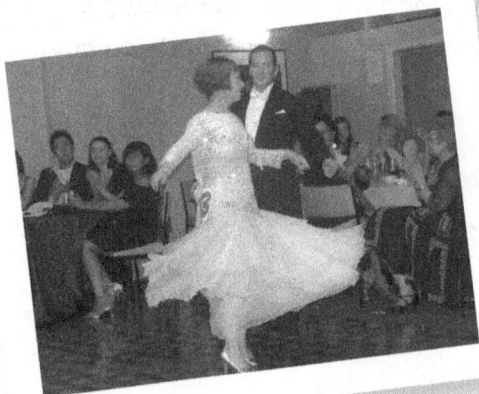

'... one of the photos was a nude shot, taken from the back. This photograph was particularly important to me. It demonstrated to me that it didn't matter that I had only one breast.'

meet Liddy Clark in Melbourne on a cold windy day and the former Queensland State Minister, actor, producer, voice coach, casting consultant, artist and former Queensland State politician brings a bubbling warmth to the afternoon. As we sit to talk, she tells me she feels a 'bit of a fraud' being interviewed as a woman who had fought breast cancer.

'I never think of myself as a breast cancer survivor. I just see it as a part of my life. I don't see myself like a Bonny Barry, a colleague in the Queensland Parliament who is going through treatments at the moment.

'I'm not one of those brave women who have gone through the hideous and painful treatments and struggled with surgery and medications. I've just lived with it as part of who I am since I was just a toddler,' she says. 'I was very young, and naivety has to be cherished. At that age you don't think of it as something life-threatening and terrible,' she admits. 'It was just part of me and my life.

'It is really my mother who was the brave one — the person who battled fear and despair for her daughter. She was the one who had to endure the treatments of her tiny little girl.

'During my life I have worked for charities supporting cancer, like *Relay for Life*, and in all that time I never told anyone, or admitted that I was a "survivor".

'It's only when we become thinkers that cancer has this frightening grip over us. But, for me, there was no emotional anguish. That's why I haven't previously said anything or put my hand up as a survivor, because it's a totally different feeling. Yes, my life is a story about getting through breast cancer, but not one of survival.'

However, Liddy's personal account shows that there is a unique story for every woman diagnosed with breast cancer. Her survival is her courage in living with the ravages that her childhood breast cancer imposed on her body.

It all began for Liddy about 51 years ago, when she was just nine months old and living in South Australia. Her two-year-old brother was just getting over polio, so when her mother noticed a growth on

Liddy's chest she became very worried about it. It was found to be a breast tumour.

'Those were the very early days of radiation treatment, and doctors were just starting to discover what could be done and beginning to understand how radiotherapy could be used in these types of situations. So I guess I was lucky that those new treatments were available — however basic they were back then.

'People talk about having flashbacks to when they were a child, and how they don't really understand them. I've had many and I also have always had problems breathing. My mother tells me that because the radiotherapy equipment was in its formative years and I was a wriggling baby, the doctors would place huge heavy weights on my chest to keep me still and to protect the rest of my body, and my mother had to keep me still. They would then put the radiation machine over that.' As Liddy recalls this, I notice one of her hands involuntarily covering her chest.

'I had that treatment for days and days and days — all these heavy weights. Then the tumour started to grow again, and the specialist said they would need to burn from underneath. My mother said the treatments were only about a minute or so at a time because I was such a tiny baby, but to her it seemed like an hour. So I think it explains my history of chest problems. As well, all my life, whenever I am nervous, I have this constricting dead-weight feeling in my chest.'

When I ask if Liddy's illness and her elder brother's polio could have been related, her face breaks into a grin. 'One of my oogly-boogly statements would be that my brother was ill and having lots of attention so, to get noticed, I got ill too. However, given the nature of the growth, that isn't realistic, is it?' she asks.

'Looking back, I realise that getting a breast tumour at that young age was unusual and I sometimes wonder if the diagnosis was totally accurate and,' she quips cheekily 'maybe they just wanted to use all of this newfangled equipment — and here I was!'

The many weeks of radiation treatment, however, did leave Liddy with a catastrophic legacy. 'I didn't know until I reached puberty that all the growth tissues had been burnt by the heavy radiation. The treatment did ensure the tumour was gone, but when I started to develop as a teenager I only grew a breast on one side. I also had an enduring radiation rash, a deep burn, on the damaged side.

'I guess it was lucky for them that it happened in the 1950s because in our now very litigious society I could have a field day with the medicos,' she adds wryly.

By this time the Clark family had moved to Melbourne. She was taken to doctors for a series of opinions. All of the doctors agreed that there were no traces of cancer, but that radiation had meant that all tissue had been destroyed.

'So I guess my story is how does a child go through the growth and development stage with the legacy of a breast tumour as a baby?'

Her mother had always said that she was pleased that it was Liddy rather than her elder sister, who was diagnosed, because she felt 'my sister would not have been able to deal with it. But because of my personality I could cope. I don't know about that — and it really did upset me every time Mum said it — but I guess the whole saga has made me who I am today.'

Her memories of those early teenage years are very different from those of most adolescent girls. She will never forget the embarrassment of being fitted for her first bra.

'It was a 30AAA, and with only one breast, you can only imagine how I felt. I always had inserts in my left side. My mother made them from bird seed and curtain weights. She also made my bathing suits, always halter-neck and also with the bird-seed inners. People now ask whether they were uncomfortable, but they were just what I knew.' It was Liddy's pragmatic approach to her situation — and her sense of humour — that saw her through this period of her life.

'Many of my school memories were also clouded with my bra mishaps, like playing chasey in the school yard and losing my false breast in various areas around the playground. But I admit that having the personality I was given meant that I was also a bit naughty with it. I remember being in sewing classes and using my left breast as a pin cushion or dramatically putting needles into my left false breast. It was long before any oil prosthesis had been invented, although I had moved to stocking inserts by the end of school.'

Whilst Liddy says that she 'just buried her physical problem', she also recognises, when reflecting on her school years, that it was probably a lot easier to handle having the operation as a toddler, rather than as a teenager or in her 20s or 30s. But she did have difficulties.

'Even the fact that my mother had to specially make all of my clothes and my bathers did make me different and did make me have to think about how I looked and presented myself.'

An example that illustrates this concern with her body image occurred after Liddy had left school and became a budding young actor. 'I had to have "composite" photos done to take around to agents. I got mine done and one of the photos was a nude shot, taken from the back. This photograph was particularly important to me. It demonstrated to me that it didn't matter that I had only one breast. Unfortunately, though, that backfired on me badly.

'Cash–Harmon Productions were auditioning for actresses for *Number 96*, one of the television soapie-style shows they were producing in the early 1970s. They saw my photo and called me in, telling me I would have to take my clothes off. I told them at the casting that it would depend on camera angles because I had only one breast. The producer was absolutely furious and screamed at me for what he called "false advertising". I told him not to worry because I was no longer interested — but it was a defining moment for me.'

However, this tough lady was not put off and in 1973 she auditioned for the one-line role of a prostitute in her first stage show, *No Sex Please, We Are British*. She got the role, and the costume designers wanted lots of cleavage for her costume. 'Well, I had to explain they could only have one-sided cleavage, and the producers again got terribly angry with me. I tried to explain that the role was about my skills not my breasts. However, to their credit, they did redesign the costume with wonderful exposure on my well-developed side and then draped a scarf over the flat side.'

Liddy then toured Australia and New Zealand in *Doctor in the House*. The larrikin in Liddy continued to put on the clown act — perhaps, she concedes, to camouflage her deeper feelings about her physical attributes.

'When we were touring in New Zealand, my party trick was that whenever we were swimming, I'd do a few laps then bounce out of the pool and, in front of everybody, I'd wring out my left breast, then go into the pool again. Appalling stuff,' she laughs, 'but probably I'd do it to prove I was okay — and possibly even to get in before anyone else,' she admits.

However, after an embarrassing leak when her oil insert dripped green dye during a performance, she decided at 22 that she would have a breast reconstruction and an inserted prosthesis.

As had been the case when she had radiotherapy, breast reconstruction was still in its early days. Unfortunately, the implant went hard the very day after her operation. 'So since then I have had a very lopsided appearance because my left breast was hard and small whilst my right side grew almost huge in comparison: so much so that I had to wear an oil prosthesis on top of the implant. And, of course, being me, I kept it there until two years ago. I would say I just couldn't be bothered. It also occurred to me that if I did have "cosmetic surgery" then I would be shallow and vain. But really, I was just too stubborn,' she says with a shrug.

'During the years when there were a lot of people suing and litigating doctors over incorrectly doing reconstructions, my brother urged me to be a part of the class action. But after 30 years I'd just got used to it.'

With humour, Liddy reflects on those 30 years, during which, whenever she had a mammogram, staff would sit her on the table and yell for everyone to come and have a look. 'I can't believe it took me 30 years to realise I was a freak,' she says, shaking her head.

'Then, in December 2004, I decided, "It's time," and I had a full reconstruction — at probably the most hideous time in my life.'

At that stage, Liddy was the Minister for Aboriginal and Torres Strait Islander Policy in the Queensland Parliament. She'd won the seat of Clayfield in the 2001 election and was re-elected and appointed to the Ministry in 2004. She had an extremely stormy 12 months as a Minister, with controversy over a staff member taking a bottle of wine into a 'dry' Indigenous community, and the issue of taking an Aboriginal activist to Palm Island just after the riots.

'I hadn't yet resigned, and just before the parliamentary Christmas break, someone saw me in the Wesley Hospital and leaked it to the press. The newspaper headlines next day screamed, 'Is there a medical problem and is she still fit to be a Minister?''

Despite her physical challenges in a world where image, beauty and perfection are fundamental to success, Liddy's acting career burgeoned. She was a part of the ABC in the halcyon days of ABC drama and education, acted in many of Hector Crawford Productions, made several movies and was a well-known theatre actor.

'I didn't think much of it because, as I've said, I just buried it. I did enjoy, though, making fun of it. It was a bit naughty of me, but I did enjoy making it hard for the boys. I remember telling and retelling the story of being in an amorous position with a boyfriend. When he took off my bra and threw it across the room it landed with an awful thud. Well, that certainly was enough to scare them off,' she laughs.

But then she becomes serious and owns up to becoming very bored with having to explain her body. 'Especially when I was dating and starting to be sexually active, so sometimes I never did bother saying anything. And you could watch them almost shudder when their hands moved across my chest and felt the missing breast. That was difficult.

'Interestingly, with all of my relationships, everyone avoided my left breast. And that is something that I have kept with me and something that I really haven't liked,' she adds sadly.

'I didn't mention it, so neither did anyone else. And probably one of my disappointments is that men didn't embrace the difference; they couldn't even talk about it. Whereas if I'd had a female partner, she would have brought my uniqueness out into the open. Women tend to be much more open and inquisitive and would want to look and touch and feel, but I think men have a fear that it is a worry for me and therefore don't broach it,' she adds insightfully.

'But even now, with all the nips and tucks in my beautiful new reconstruction, I still don't have a nipple on one breast or feeling in the other. But, whatever — who really cares now? These days, it's from the neck up — that's the best bit of excitement now.'

Liddy's gaze meets mine, and I am struck anew by her vitality.

And with that she wraps her bright emerald sweater around the two now pert breasts and rushes off to her ballroom dancing class. She looks far removed from the self-proclaimed freak and more like a fabulous breast cancer survivor who has really twirled and danced her way through life.

Hello Beautiful FOAM Friends

Well, today I finally did it. Ross Coco shaved my head. And really, underneath that spunky blonde hair was a rather attractive head — no big bumps or lumps or scars and, according to some, quite a shapely cranium!

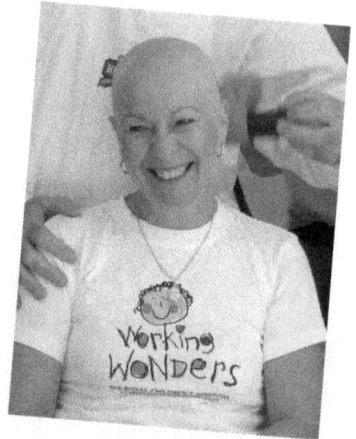

That's the physical side. The emotional side is a whole different kettle of fish. Once I decided to have my head shaved for charity, I probably experienced the whole range of emotions on whatever is the bald equivalent of the Richter Scale. One moment I am delighting in the feeling of empowerment — of taking control of my own future and being able to make a small community contribution. (One of the producers at 4BC, who has the most amazingly flamboyant curly long hair, told me when she was 21 and in London she shaved her head. She said she felt totally liberated and wonderfully free.) That gave me courage and motivation. I was ready to face the world boldly like Zena of Freshwater — then the next minute, I am flooded with tears knowing that my hair is one of my signatures and wondering if my self-esteem and my identity will tumble along with my locks.

Deep down I knew I was doing the right thing, but when people kept telling me I didn't have to do it and to only shave if it was for me, I was catapulted into uncertainty.

Well, it's done and I have had my first public outing — to the Coles supermarket in New Farm. Okay, so it is a mecca for the wonderfully beautiful A-listers, but there are enough 'individuals' in the area to make me feel brave enough to venture forth.

Reality really hit. I lined up at the checkout, with pumpkin, cashews, milk and toilet paper under my arm, at the busiest supermarket around and heard a little girl's voice very loudly say, 'Hey, lady, have you got cancer?' You could hear a pin drop in Coles. I looked around to see a 5 or 6-year-old little girl in pink looking at me. I was very embarrassed, but looking into her eyes I realised that there was no animosity or vindictiveness — she just wanted to know. So I said to her, 'Yes, I have. How did you know?' to which she replied, 'Silly. You've got a cancer head.'

Yep, I do have a cancer head, and it took the innocent curiosity of a tot to make me realise that it was going to be tough — but I would be okay.

Later that night, seeing my image reflected back on the television news was also very daunting. But, hey! This is me for the next little while. My soul and spirit are still the same — although maybe a little richer for the experience. My hair will grow back and I only hope that it isn't bright red and frizzy!!!! (Apologies to anyone with that combination ... on you, it looks lovely!)

When I go out tomorrow and to work on Monday, it will be the same me — just a little less hairy and with no need of gel.

Smile

AM

Elissa MacLeod's Journey

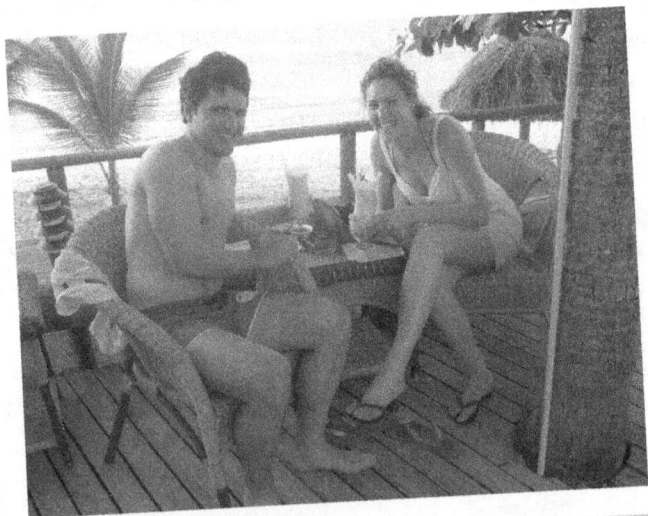

'I don't think any of us knew how to handle it, who to tell and how to tell people. I was adamant I didn't want people, especially boys, to pity me or even look at me as if I wasn't attractive.'

I first met Elissa MacLeod in Brisbane in 2007 when she was playing National League Netball with the Melbourne Kestrels against the Queensland Firebirds. I was organising the media for the match and when I talked briefly with Elissa, little did I know we had more in common than a passion for netball.

We had both heard those terrible words, 'I am sorry, you have breast cancer.'

Catching up again with the striking blonde, now a businesswoman in Melbourne, gave me an insight into the amazing courage and fortitude of Elissa MacLeod.

Elissa's journey with cancer began in 2003. She was only 19 years old when she first noticed an unusual lump in her breast. She didn't really know what to do about it, and as she is a very private person, talking about the lump to anyone was 'a big deal for me'.

Then, a little while after this discovery, Elissa had a spell of vertigo; she couldn't move and every time she got up the world was spinning. 'So because we didn't know what was wrong with me, Mum took me off to hospital,' explains Elissa.

'I had told Mum about the lump but I couldn't tell anyone else. So, as I was in hospital I asked the doctor to check it out for me. The doctor told me I was too young for it to be anything sinister and the lump was just normal young fibrous tissue and that I would be fine. I thought, "Well, that's it and I don't need to worry." But I was feeling very ill-at-ease as he was checking the lump and right back then, I had a niggling sense that everything actually wasn't fine.'

Two years later Elissa was selected in the Victorian Under-21 team to compete in the Australian National Netball titles in Canberra in September 2005. In spite of being reassured, she was worried about the lump. 'It hadn't gone away and although I continued to monitor it, I just felt it shouldn't be still there.

'Just before leaving for the Championships, I told my mum that I was concerned about it and that when I got back I'd get it checked out again,' says Elissa.

'Then just before the first game at the Nationals, I found bloodstains in my bra from a discharge from my nipple in that same breast. It was from this moment I knew my instincts were correct and the lump was not "normal". This discharge confirmed what I had always known — that everything was not okay.

'I didn't think it was breast cancer, but I knew there was something wrong and I never really let it go. I thought maybe it was a cyst, but when I was diagnosed with breast cancer, having had a sense something was wrong didn't diminish the shock of diagnosis,' she says.

I notice a faraway look in Elissa's eyes as she casts her mind back. A slight shadow flickers across her features.

'I was immediately snuck away by the team manager to the hospital to get the lump checked in between games, and to make sure I was okay to play. The doctor was again not overly concerned, considering I had no breast cancer family history and I was so young. But he gave me a referral to have a mammogram when I got back to Melbourne.

'I played the rest of the Nationals — some of the best netball I had ever played in centre position — but in my head I was awaiting the return to Melbourne, and anticipating what would happen over the next few weeks.

'I didn't tell anyone except my best friend, Chelsey Nash. I wanted to keep it to myself and I also thought that the team, although they were my friends, were too young to have to deal with this.'

The day Elissa got back to Melbourne she went straight in to have a mammogram. Immediately following that, the radiologist performed an ultrasound. 'Then they asked me if I had a specialist that I could see. A specialist? I didn't, and still don't even have a GP, so they quickly sent me upstairs to see the oncologist.

'He then organised for me to have numerous biopsies.' And then she laughs as she says, 'They really have to do something about the loud noise those machines make as they take a sample of your tissue!

'All of this immediate attention should have been a hint, and although I always had a gut instinct that there was something wrong, I never believed breast cancer was on the horizon.

'The findings were at first unconvincing. I was really impressed with the persistent efforts from my amazing oncologist, Craig Murphy, who was not prepared to settle for those inconclusive results. To find the definitive diagnosis, I finally had an operation to remove a larger sample of tissue.

'Finally,' says Elissa, 'the results came in: ductal carcinoma in situ — pre-cancer cells that will at any stage become cancerous. It was a very large lump and there were areas of calcification that were really spread throughout that breast.'

When I ask Elissa about her feelings and the devastation this diagnosis must have caused she stuns me with her grateful and positive outlook.

'What did I think? Well, how lucky that I had a discharge that brought enough attention to that lump so that I required further examination. How lucky I had a doctor who insisted on having conclusive results and looked further than most would. How lucky that I was *not* sick. How lucky that I had the option to do something to stop myself getting sick. How lucky — in the event I would lose my breast — that a reconstruction was possible!

'Dr Craig Murphy's strong advice was for a mastectomy, and he reeled off the percentage rates of a cancer reoccurrence if you had a mastectomy, a lumpectomy or just radiotherapy. I can't remember the exact figures but it seemed like only 2 per cent if I had a mastectomy. You can't argue with that.

'I know lots of women have great trouble making that decision, but for me it was very obvious that a mastectomy was the best option. Obviously, this was a very regretful decision as I had great young boobs,' she laughs. 'Ideally, I would have never considered losing one of my breasts, but the choice was never hard. It was always a no-brainer. How couldn't I give myself the highest percentage chance of not getting cancer and not getting sick? So this is what was meant to happen, and I was going to deal with it.'

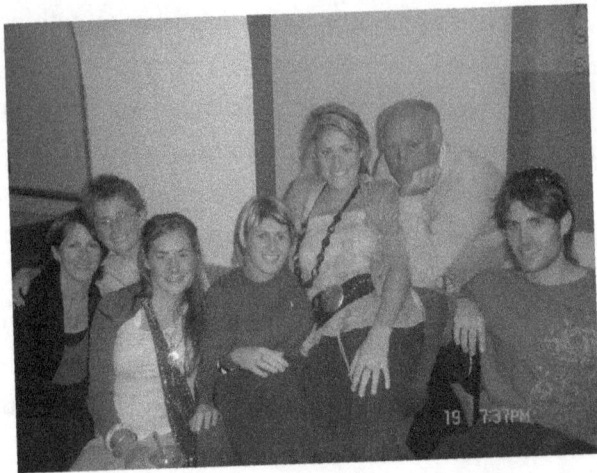

Elissa with her family gathered around her

Whilst Elissa's decision was straightforward for her, some friends and other women she has since talked with have wondered about her medical assessment and the choice she made.

'I was talking with another young breast cancer survivor a little while ago. She was 27, and her doctors discouraged her from having a mastectomy at such a young age. I don't know why. Maybe my doctor thought that I was strong and mature enough to emotionally and physically cope with such a drastic choice.'

The decision was not taken lightly by Elissa, her parents, Jenny and John, or her medical team. All of her tests and samples were sent to the United Kingdom to double-check the results. 'I guess the doctors just wanted to make absolutely sure. Cutting off a 21-year-old girl's breast is rather dramatic, and the doctors were just triple-checking.'

When Elissa was initially told it was cancer, she says everything stopped in the world. 'I went white and even though I am a big thinker, at that moment there were no thoughts in my head: everything went completely blank. I remember Mum was crying, and all I could do was stare at the doctor. When the doctor asked if I was okay, I was startled back into life and immediately began thinking about what I needed to do.'

One of the first questions Elissa asked was about the cost of the treatments. 'We are not a really wealthy family and straight away I was anxious that my parents would have to fork out money that they could spend in other ways. Of course, Mum told me not to worry. The doctors gave me pamphlets with scary pictures. I worried about my boyfriend and how he would cope. It was all overwhelming and yet I needed to know what had to be done so I could get organised.'

Elissa tells me that when she and her mother walked out of the surgeon's room, she burst into tears as she prepared to ring her longtime boyfriend, Andrew. 'I was so confused and upset trying to tell Andrew what was happening. I couldn't say the word "mastectomy". I'd never ever used that word before, and it is such a horrible, negative word that it was absolutely terrible trying to explain the significance of the diagnosis and the serious implications of it all to Andrew. It was so tough.'

Surprisingly, Elissa never really thought of the diagnosis as a death sentence, as so many do at that moment. 'No, I never thought I would die. Because we had caught it so early and it was pre-cancer cells, I felt I would get through. I felt so lucky that we had found it before it developed into cancer and it spread; before death was in the equation.'

'When we left the doctor's surgery, we met my dad and I told my best friend, Chelsey, and so I had to go through it all again. But I also decided not to tell many people. We were such a young family and I didn't know how to act about it. I don't think any of us knew how to handle it, who to tell and how to tell people. I was adamant I didn't want people — especially boys — to pity me or even look at me as if I wasn't attractive,' she admits.

'I didn't want the sympathy vote and even at that age I didn't want other girls to feel I had a compassionate advantage. Silly, I know, but these are the things that ran through my perhaps irrational brain in those early days.

'I didn't want pity and I certainly didn't want people to be disgusted. I guess I was a little ashamed. I don't really know why. If I am thinking realistically I know there is no reason to think like that. I don't want people to feel bad for me because I don't feel bad for myself.'

She recalls one incident from those early days that stands out in her memory. 'I made the mistake of telling a school friend about the cancer and she reacted very badly. I was telling her I couldn't go to her birthday party and she couldn't understand why. So I told her I had early breast cancer and she just got angry at me and didn't know what to say or do. It was unbearably uncomfortable. So I think that day also shaped my decision not to tell many people.

'Another reason is probably because I was an elite athlete and I couldn't take people seeing weakness in me. I liked it that at netball no one knew about the cancer and just treated me as a normal person. I didn't want to be defined as the netballer with cancer. I wanted to be seen and accepted as myself. I wanted to feel that my cancer was irrelevant to my ability in sport or my popularity.

'In fact, it makes me feel strong knowing that I have this little card up my sleeve — one that means I am resilient and tough. Even now, a few years later, most people I mix with have no idea I had breast cancer and so when my life has its tough moments, I can draw on that ace up my sleeve and do things I would normally have baulked at — like speaking in public!' confesses Elissa.

When diagnosed, Elissa also went through a time of confusion. 'Although I didn't consider breast cancer only as an older woman's disease, I did feel different. I was barely into my 20s. I never really questioned why it happened, because I know bad things happen to people every day. I remember thinking that I still have my teeth so I can smile; no one can see under my top to see any disfigurement; all my family is well and I am not dead. So I am very lucky,' she says.

There is a brief pause in the conversation and I am struck that Elissa possesses wisdom and maturity beyond her years. It also occurs to me that playing netball so well while waiting to have surgery for cancer must have seemed an incredible paradox.

Once Elissa was ready for surgery she took advice to have the mastectomy and reconstruction in the one operation.

'Again, I think that decision was because of my youth. All through this time I felt I was always treated as a special patient. I know the doctors are always very attentive, but I suspect my age made me a little special in their eyes. What could have been absolutely horrific turned out to be okay.'

Elissa's mastectomy and reconstruction was booked for the week before Christmas 2006. This period was a turning point in her life — not only was she having surgery to protect herself from breast cancer, but she would also need to take time to evaluate her future life.

'When I got back from the 2005 Netball Nationals I had been very pleased with my performances on court. In fact, the Australian coach, Norma Plummer, had commented on how well I had played, which was exciting for me,' Elissa tells me.

Other coaches had also identified Elissa's talent on court and she was asked to trial for the Melbourne Kestrels team.

'I had already had arthroscopy on my dodgy netball knee whilst I was dealing with all the breast cancer stuff, but I was really keen to keep playing netball and pursuing a normal active life. I told the coach I had "other stuff" going on in my life, but I was desperate to be considered. I told her if I was picked I would get my knee fixed immediately as the arthroscope had shown my knee needed surgery. The sore knee and the affected breast were both on the left side and I wondered what was going on with my body,' Elissa admits.

As an aside, Elissa mentions that she was having reiki treatments to help her through the stress of her breast cancer diagnosis. On one occasion she was treated by a reiki practitioner who also practised sports reiki — 'and after that session I haven't had one bit of trouble from my knee, and I had been struggling with it since I was 16,' says Elissa, stretching out the knee in question. 'Believe it or not, I just know my knee was fixed and I went back to top-level netball.'

Elissa didn't make the Kestrels team that year, but played impressively enough in State league to be selected in 2007 into

Kestrels. 'That was an awesome reward for all the hard work and for my determination to recover from all the tough stuff in my life the previous year. The bonus was that Chelsey captained the team and life was very sweet,' says Elissa proudly.

The following year Kestrels was disbanded as netball moved into the new international ANZ Championship competition. This gave Elissa the opportunity to broaden her netball career and she was offered a contract to play in the English netball league with Team Northumbria, based in Newcastle.

'This was a wonderful break for me. I had put the cancer behind me and I was touring and travelling and having great fun playing netball at the English club's expense. It was a dream and I grabbed it eagerly.'

Elissa is now back playing as captain–coach of the Melbourne University team in the premier league in Victoria — just for fun and to keep fit.

Elissa's belief in living the best life she can and being grateful she has that opportunity is one of the defining features of her story. Her close relationships with friends and family throughout her life — especially during the testing times of 2005 — are also significant for her.

'Family and close friends are the most important part of my life. Throughout my journey they have been there beside me. When I woke up in hospital after my surgery, Chelsey had decorated my whole room with a chain of stars she hand-made, which brightened up my room.'

Elissa looks back fondly at her time in hospital, recovering from her operation in a room full of balloons, motivational pictures, notes, flowers.

'How could I not be happy when I woke up to that joy? Chelsey has been there from when I first thought I had something wrong and is still my best friend — she is an angel.'

Also at her side for the entire journey has been her boyfriend, Andrew. 'He stood by me the whole way. He will say he hasn't done anything special and that "I am just Andrew and you are just Elissa" and nothing will ever change that. Having my breast removed hasn't seemed to change anything for him — and, to a certain extent, why should it? He is right — I am still Elissa. He never shied away from me or felt I was anyone different because of what I went through. He never really did anything that was amazing or tried to smooth things over. He was just there — and there all of the time.

'He came to all the medical appointments with me and my family. The best thing was we just did normal things like playing rock, scissors, paper in the waiting room. He never ran away when things were difficult. He kept me normal,' Elissa says with a shrug and a glowing smile.

I ask Elissa what impact her cancer — and the necessity of dealing with such a confronting emotional and physical ordeal at such a young and very vulnerable age — has had on her attitude and the way she looks at life.

'Having breast cancer didn't really change me, but it did give me the opportunity to be the *real me*. I already knew I was strong, I already knew I thought of myself as more than just my looks and my body. So the cancer gave me the chance to be true to myself — to be Elissa.

'Does it change what I do today? No. But it sometimes does make me more aware of myself and my body. For instance, when I get tired I get really upset about being tired and maybe worry too much about it. Then I know I need to slow down and look after myself.

'Do I worry that perhaps the cancer will come back? I didn't think about it at all for a while but in the past two years I regularly check my other breast for lumps. A little while ago I found a small lump and I was really scared. But my oncologist got me in the next day and found it was just hormonal. I do worry about secondary cancer — that's what you die from,' she admits. 'More recently the thought of children and my ability to breastfeed comes into my mind. I sometimes worry that I may be plagued with hormonal problems — but that is for the future.'

Since the mastectomy three years ago, Elissa has had regular aesthetic operations on her reconstructed breast. 'I've had to go into hospital seven times. When I first had the operation the plastic surgeon used a silicone implant and my muscle to give the new breast its shape. I was so fit at the time that I didn't have any fat on my stomach for the doctors to transpose to my breast. They were worried that if they took the muscles and fat from this area, that I may have problems when I had children. But because I am so sporty, the muscles in the implant get distorted. So now they are going to inject fat from my stomach every three months for this coming year,' she explains.

'I am so lucky to have the best plastic surgeon in the world. Professor Ashton is so good to me, and is happy to persist at creating for me the very best breast that he can.'

She then goes on to tell the tale of misconceptions during one of these operations. 'It is very daunting fronting up for the operations and as I am really very shy I always wear a singlet. This particular time I had an older anaesthetist. He pulled down my gown roughly and I could feel from the way he looked at me that he was judging me. He obviously thought I was a young girl willing to undergo cosmetic surgery in order to have fashionable breasts and he certainly didn't approve.

'Then in walked Professor Ashton, who introduced me and explained I was "their special breast cancer patient". Well, the anaesthetist was certainly mortified and his manner improved immediately. I get very angry with people who judge me,' she says strongly. 'He thought I was shallow, and I am not shallow so it really annoyed me.'

Throughout our interview, Elissa struggled each time she mentioned the words 'breast cancer'. When I ask her about this, she confesses that she still struggles to use those words. 'Yes, I guess I find it really difficult and until I began doing awareness speeches I never said I'd had breast cancer. I guess because I had pre-cancer I never actually had cancer. I thought that I'd escaped it and I didn't want to make a

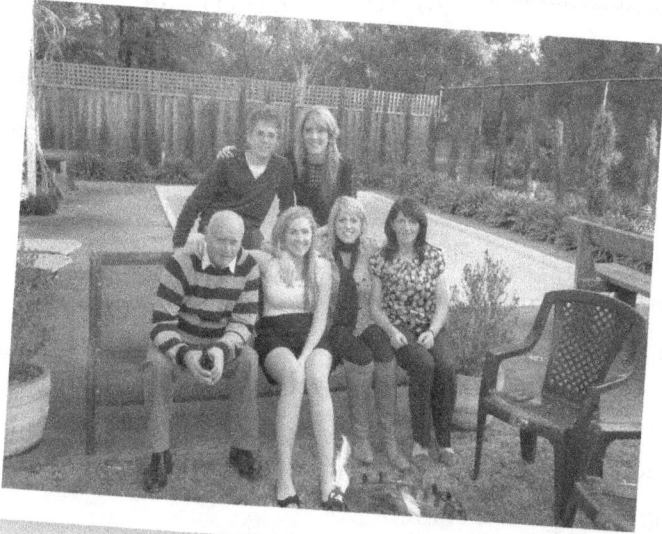

The MacLeod clan (Elissa at rear)

fuss. In hindsight, I should have made more of a fuss and been more proud of myself and the way I've handled myself,' explains Elissa.

In spite of Elissa's humility and shyness in talking about her breast cancer journey she feels extremely strongly about making other women, in particular very young women, very aware about the reality of breast cancer. Her cancer has influenced her to make a difference.

'I approached the National Breast Cancer Foundation because I realised I had a story that could be of use to them — for a few reasons. I wanted to alert people so they could get to the cancer before they got sick, no matter how old they were. I also appreciated the tremendous support I received through my illness so I wanted to thank those people, but I also wanted to encourage people in general to look after those in need. Finally, I thought people may be able to draw strength from my story. I hope that just maybe I can inspire people going through breast cancer treatment, or young people or women in general with body image issues. If me telling my story helps just one person, then my mission is complete,' says Elissa.

Looking ahead, Elissa is excited about her future — and especially about the fact that she has one. 'I want to do some more travel, have lots of babies, be rich and hopefully get a big diamond ring!' she says with a twinkle in her eye. 'Some days my journey makes me impatient and want more from life, and I start to believe I could do anything — be the first female prime minister, a CEO of a global company. Other days I am just happy looking outside and seeing the world for what it is and being very ordinary.

'At the time I was diagnosed I felt very strongly that there was a reason for my journey with breast cancer. In fact, I remember the reiki guy telling me he felt I had a big purpose in life. Sometimes I think I was given cancer young because I could deal with it and then stand up and raise awareness.'

And as this stunning young woman, who has so captivated my heart and inspired me, stands up to go back to work, she leans over and says in a conspiratorial whisper, 'There are a few moments in my journey with breast cancer that are a personal victory for me. No one knows about my cancer. A guy walked past me on the street on my way here and had a little perve at my breasts. I smiled back thinking, "If only you knew what was down there."

From: AnneMarie

Subject: DAYS OF OUR LIVES OR THE BALD
AND BEAUTIFUL?

Sent: 20 August 2003

No: It's The Bald and Beautiful and Bilious!

Hello again dear FOAM friends

The past week has been an interesting experience — having
gone bald quickly and publicly, I had to learn about going out
in public without the Being Bald 101 and 102 lectures.

Also I have solved the foundation question — just on the
nose and then big eyes and big smiley lippie — oh and lots of
courage!!!!

Chemo Number 4.

This was the chemo that was going to go perfectly. I leave
tomorrow morning at sparrow twitter to drive with Pete
to Canberra to visit with Nessie. I haven't seen my bestest
daughter since she came up in May when I was diagnosed
with cancer. Although we talk almost every day and I send
regular pics, it is not the same at all. I can't wait to just hug
her and tell her everything — the good and the yukky, but
mostly that I am going fine and that I love her! Remember
the song 'In the Living Years'? I need to do that lots lately.

So for the preceding week I went off the alcohol, onto juices,
lots of good healthy food and running each morning and

even early nights!! So I lined up very happy and confident on Monday morning.

Everything went well, my neutrophils were terrific and my white blood cells were great too. Chemo went smoothly and Pete took me home. At 5.30 I'm feeling terrific and smirking about how easy it was. At 6 I sit down to watch the news and the old stomach is a little rumbly and by 6.15 I'm in the bathroom sick again.

I take my oncologist's full emergency pack and am okay for another hour but then after dropping another internal load I'm off to hospital once again.

Emergency is a riot, with lots of people ill and too few nurses, and doctors who are really struggling to do their caring best with the huge crowd. Eventually I get a drip and my anti-nausea drugs, but they don't really kick in until after midnight. The health crisis in bed shortages is real — I know — and finally, at 5am, I get a bed in the oncology ward. Because the reactions are getting worse (the build-up of chemo drugs and the slow destruction of tissues) it meant I had to stay in for three nights, hence just arriving home now.

There were moments in Emergency, lurching into bowl after bowl, where I felt it is just too much to bear and the tears started to flow. But the reality for me is that this is my choice. I chose to have chemo as an insurance against reoccurrence and so the big picture is that these are the yukky down times, but they are balanced by the wonderful moments along my journey — the gift of friendships by so many gorgeous people, the prayers of people I know and even those I hardly know. Books, food, juices, flowers, hugs and touching emails. Who could ask for anything more?

Pete and I leave tomorrow for Canberra and Vanesa, and we will be home officially on September 1st after a few days at the farm. Spring!! Yeah. September is also when my brand new grandchild is due.

I know why I'm coping during these bad days when I think of the ab fab days of kids, grandkids and friends ... especially my FOAMs.

Love you all very much. Thank you for being there for me.

AM

Daphne Pirie's Journey

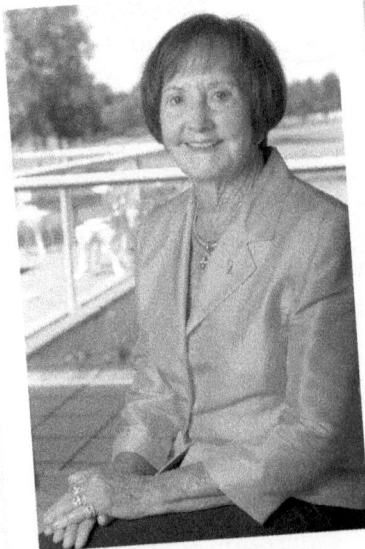

*'Right from the beginning I never thought I was going to die —
but then again, I never really dwelt on such a morbid subject.
I had confidence I would get over it quickly, but I was too smart
for myself and it hasn't been quick.'*

There is no other way of introducing her: Daphne Pirie is a dynamo. At 77 years of age, her enthusiasm for living a full and useful life and her optimistic outlook is incredible. Just sitting talking to her is inspiring and she fills me with awe.

In her younger days, Daphne was an international athlete: a champion sprinter — running alongside Marjorie Jackson, Shirley Strickland and Marlene Mathews — and an Australian hockey player. Her dedication to sport, from the grass-roots level to the ultimate elite, the Olympics, has been acknowledged with many national honours.

When she turned 50, Daphne began an illustrious career as a Masters athlete and held eight world records in sprints and high jump. She was a popular competitor and an international champion who commanded respect throughout the world.

When Daphne was diagnosed with breast cancer in November 2006 she adopted the same fierce champion attitude to beating the illness as she had to crushing her opposition on the tartan track. 'I knew how to win as an athlete and I was going to use every one of those skills to beat this disease.' She has held this attitude, which she adopted straight after her diagnosis, throughout her journey. Daphne is a warrior sportswoman, and she is determined to win this battle.

Daphne learned at a very young age how to be positive and make the most of life. She credits her optimistic outlook in the face of the terrors of cancer to her parents' influence. 'I grew up in a family of ten and so I learned at a very young age how to be positive. I learned if I was to achieve and get through then I would have to work hard. The same principles apply for me in any challenge — whether it be sport or life or my health. Being diagnosed with breast cancer was just one more test,' she says.

Her diagnosis came as a sudden and unexpected shock. 'I found a small lump in my breast and immediately I had to face reality — I wasn't indestructible. But I struggled to accept that I had breast cancer.

'I remember feeling cold and shocked — as most women must do when they find a lump. It was very, very small and right up into my armpit. The timing wasn't very good — although I guess it never is. Sadly, at that time my husband, Mick, had had a heart problem and he was in hospital having a mitral valve replaced. Our two sons were beside themselves with worry about their father, so I just kept this news to myself,' she says.

Daphne quickly took herself off to her gynaecologist in the hope that the lump was just a cyst and nothing to be concerned about. She says that she was too busy looking after Mick to have time to think about herself and what might potentially be a major health problem for her.

She had a mammogram and a few days later, while driving along the highway on her way home, she got a phone call from her doctor. 'I knew it was bad because he told me to pull off the road. He then told me that the mammogram and ultrasound had shown cancer cells and that I should get myself off to hospital straight away.

'But I couldn't do that because Mick was still in intensive care and I needed to be there for him. So I put it off for a couple of weeks. I honestly believed that there was nothing wrong with me, and I was so concerned about Mick that in the big scheme of things it didn't seem like I needed to rush,' she replies calmly.

Eventually Daphne did consult specialists, who diagnosed cancer, and she had a lumpectomy. At that stage, she felt, in her pragmatic way, that she was fine and could get back to looking after Mick during his convalescence. But cancer cells had been detected in six lymph nodes and she was told that she would need a full auxiliary clearance. Further tests revealed that there were three breast cancer cells and three lymphoma cells.

'This was very unusual. Usually, lymphoma is somewhere else, but I had both cancers in cells in my lymph nodes. My breast cancer doctor was very surprised and hadn't expected them at all.

'Now, that really worried me. I didn't know much about breast cancer before this, but I had noticed a lady at our golf club who had a thick arm from the disease. So it terrified me that I might get a swollen arm and not be able to play sport any more. Funnily enough,

I wasn't worried about dying, just about not being able to play golf or run.

'As I was waiting before I went back into the operating theatre, I said to the nurse, "I think I'll split because I can't cope with this." But she told me it would be very foolish. I already knew that. I was just very scared. So I went ahead and had the clearance operation done.

'The nurses told me later that even while I was in the recovery room, I was trying to lift my arm to see if it still worked properly,' she laughs. 'That operation worried me much more than the first one — especially as I now seemed to be dealing with two very different types of cancer in my body. My biggest problem was getting all the information clear in my mind, because each specialist would only talk about his own cancer area. I know they talked to each other, but I found it hard to get the overall picture,' says Daphne with a shake of her head.

When diagnosed, some women dive into information overload, researching the disease and all its implications on the 'net, and reading as many books as they can get their hands on so they feel they know everything about the disease. Daphne, on the other hand, decided to put her full trust in the professionalism of her large medical team.

'When the doctors told me that I had two types of cancer simultaneously, I was in a bit of a spin. It was all too confusing and complicated for me. But talking individually with each of the doctors, and knowing that they also regularly consulted with each other on my case, I knew that everything they did would be in my best interests. As an athlete, I always listened to my coaches, my nutritionists and all the support staff. I knew they had the expertise and knowledge to make me the best athlete I could be. So I decided from the beginning it was best to just follow the doctors' advice,' says Daphne.

She was now dealing with non-Hodgkins lymphoma — a type of leukaemia of the blood — as well as breast cancer. Each cancer would need to be treated both in isolation and with reference to the other. Treating the breast cancer was always going to be the priority, but because of the complications of lymphoma, it was several weeks before her medical team worked out a plan for Daphne's care.

'I needed chemotherapy for each of the cancers, but different types for each one. I had chemotherapy to target the breast cancer, but with an addition of Vincristine for the lymphoma. Then I had heart tests to make sure I was strong enough to be able to take the chemo mixture.'

Daphne struggled a little with all the attention of doctors and medical specialists. 'I didn't want any fuss. I went to all the appointments by myself and tried to stay as private as I possibly could. I really felt embarrassed to be sick. I'd always been the picture of good health and suddenly here I am — a sick old lady. I was very worried about my image. Right from when I was young my father impressed upon me that it was important what other people thought of you, and I thought all my colleagues — especially in the world of sport — would judge me. With my poor health, I worried that maybe it wouldn't look right for me to be working on boards, especially with elite athletes. At the root of it, I guess I was just so embarrassed not to be perfectly fit and healthy,' admits Daphne.

'Pride isn't such a good thing, is it?' she asks me. 'But it was a very humbling experience. It was a big learning curve and I know I have come out of this a better person.'

Daphne has friends who had been diagnosed with cancer and had decided not to go through chemotherapy. However, Daphne reasoned that if chemo was going to help her get rid of the cancers, then she would take her doctors' advice and go through with it.

With her very positive attitude, Daphne would have her regular chemo sessions and then 'I'd put on my neck-to-knees swimmers and head for the beach. I loved the feeling of the salt water cleansing me. My hair fell out almost immediately and I carefully exposed my bald head at the beach to a little sun — as my daily Vitamin D supplement!' she laughs.

In her sporting days Daphne had been known as the 'Flying Redhead', a reference to her distinctive dark red hair. 'Now,' she laughs again, 'that red hair was flying out the window! I didn't really mind the loss of my hair, but I hated wearing wigs and hats and only did so when I had to.'

Once chemo was finished, Daphne undertook a course of radiation therapy. 'The funny thing about this treatment was that I knew it wouldn't hurt and that once I'd done the chemo, nothing could be as bad. But I needed to hang on to some independence going through it. I guess it was my sporting discipline that insisted that if I was going to win, I needed to be in control of myself. So I drove myself down the coast every day for treatment, and counted off the treatments day by day. I also believed that if I felt I was well enough to drive, then I was going to be okay. So my independence was really my way of convincing myself that I would get better.'

Just prior to finishing the radiation, in June 2007, she was feeling quite positive about her future but was curious about what impact the drugs had had on her body. So Daphne went to her local sports doctor for a check-up. He did a series of tests and, after he viewed the results, expressed concern about her heart, telling Daphne she needed to go to a heart specialist straight away. 'I just gasped and said, "No way." I already had a battery of doctors, I didn't need any more. By this stage, my husband had recovered from his heart surgery, but was due for a check-up. So I gave Mick my cardiology print-out and asked him to see what his cardiologist thought.'

Much to her surprise and dismay, Daphne's heart had gone into an irregular rhythm and she had a leaking valve. 'I was devastated, and still find it hard to believe. As well as the two cancers, I now had atrial fibrillation. This meant I had to go onto Warfarin and eight other tablets for ever to regulate my dicky heart. That's when my body started to rebel and my life changed. My heart doctor is convinced the chemo caused the changes, although my oncologist isn't so sure. The bottom line is that I now had a major setback with my heart and I just had to deal with it.

'The problems with my heart posed a challenge for me. Maybe because I'm an athlete, I have always had very low blood pressure, but the tablets I had to take lowered it even further. I have collapsed a few times and ended up in hospital, which I hate.' As she says this, I register Daphne's sigh of frustration. 'I hate having these tablets because I've always resisted putting poisons in my body — even when I was going through chemo I didn't take any additional medications. But this time I knew that without them I would die.'

The good news for Daphne was that her mammograms post-treatment were clear. So this feisty woman decided that she had had enough of being a patient. 'I was feeling good and I wanted to get my life back, so I went back to golf. I am very competitive and it was exciting to be playing again. I played 18 holes in a competition and really played hard and won. But two days later I discovered that I had a massive infection in my breast, spreading throughout my chest. I realised that because I didn't have any lymph glands under my driving arm, with the pressure of playing energetically, I had created scar tissue bleeding, which had drained into my breast.

'In normal circumstances this would have been easy to treat with antibiotics, but because of my heart problems I had to have even more tests before they could fix me. With the infection I also had to postpone my scans for the lymphoma and my heart tests. That's what I find difficult to cope with. My life has changed; and whereas before I was never sick — and if I had something wrong with me I always healed really quickly — now everything is such a drama. And I certainly struggled to accept the weakness.

'In the beginning, the doctors' priority was treating the breast cancer and then the lymphoma, but because of the complications, my heart treatment is now controlling my life. I only feel half the person I used to be. In the past, if I saw steps I'd run up them as a bonus bit of training. Now I can barely walk up stairs at all. I am tired all the time because of the heart medications. But I had no option. If I didn't take them, I'd die — and that's not an option!' she says purposefully.

'I continued to have problems. Initially the cardiologist wouldn't let me take Arimidex for my ongoing breast cancer protection, but I

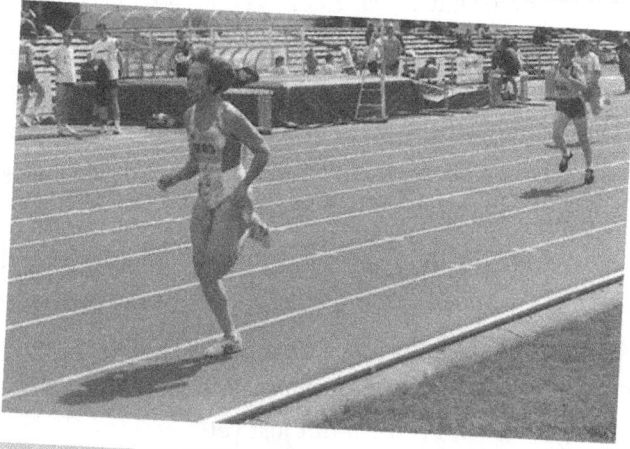

World champion Daphne, with red hair flying

was so scared of not safeguarding myself against breast cancer that I just took it — and continue to take it.

'With the lymphoma I was told I would need a bone marrow harvest, but that meant more chemo which I really didn't want to do as I felt it would play havoc with my heart again. So the doctors decided to do a maintenance treatment, a MabThera infusion, which had a similar effect to chemo in keeping the white blood count up and building my immunity, but without the side effects,' she explains. This treatment will continue every three months for two years.

So in maintenance mode, Daphne faces a far different life than she had ever imagined just two years before. 'The doctors have told me that my heart won't come good again, but I can live with that. I won't live the sort of life I wanted; however, I know I am lucky that I had already had the surgery, then chemo and radiation treatment, so when the heart problems arose it was really just another hurdle I had to face.

'I was quite certain I could still live an enjoyable life. I could never say I was in remission. What I would say is that I am living the best life I can. In fact, now I am so busy living that I don't have time to worry about what might happen,' she laughs

'I truly believed that a healthy mind created a healthy body and that I would have been able to think myself healthy. I thought that this little hiccup would be over in six months. But each day I am grateful that the cancer only struck me when I was 75. I've had a wonderful life and so today I can accept what has happened to me. I accept that this is me now.'

Looking to the future, Daphne sees a very different lifestyle from the one she had envisaged. 'I thought at 80 years old I would be training hard in athletics and hopefully travelling the world, continuing to set world records and win championships.' With a glint in her eye she adds, 'Although I haven't ruled it out just yet!

'I have had to accept a lesser lifestyle for my future. Having said that, I am very grateful that there is a future. At the beginning, the cardiologist was treating me day by day and I am sure he didn't think I'd get through. Whereas he now tells me that I am going to be great in ten years' time. That gives me confidence.' There is a real glint in Daphne's eye as she says this. She may be in her seventies but she has the sparkle and downright cheeky air of someone in their twenties.

'Funnily enough, a young friend of mine was recently enquiring about my health and she asked me if it was just old age that was the problem now. Well, that was like a red rag to a bull for me. But it did make me realise the toll the cancer has taken on me. I've gone from being in the highest level of fitness down to the lowest level.'

Daphne's amazing resilience has always been one of her personal strengths, and with all that this disease has thrown at her over the past few years, there is still not one iota of bitterness. 'No time or energy for bitterness,' she says philosophically. 'I was always intent on getting it all behind me. I also didn't want to worry my family. I didn't want them — or anyone else for that matter — to see me down and I didn't want to be a burden for them. I guess it is that old thing of pride again. Maybe that's not the right attitude, but I have always been independent and if you are, then you just can't bellyache because no one listens. I just get on with life.

'I have so many wonderful friends who want to help, but my self-sufficiency doesn't allow me to ask for assistance unless I am absolutely desperate — and I will never be desperate,' she says with a steely grin. 'I guess I've always felt that my illness was my problem and I would handle it myself in my own way — in private. Mick and the boys were supportive, although they were perhaps too easily reassured I was fine,' she laughs. 'I felt I couldn't let anyone down and so I probably downplayed my situation.'

Daphne has always seen her battle with cancer as 'one more race I had to run. And, like any other event, I trained hard for it. I was especially vigilant about my nutrition and I think that discipline again helped me deal with cancer. I juiced and ate lots of healthy fruit and vegetables. I walked and exercised whenever I was able,' she says.

'I had never thought that these treatments would go on any longer than 12 months but now I realise I am having to live a completely new lifestyle. I am pretty disappointed that my life has turned out this way because I am nervous that I could all too easily slot into an inactive, over-comfortable way of living. That is not me and I don't want to fall into that trap. I am actually frightened of being sedentary — almost dormant.'

Daphne tells me how swimming and water workouts have always been a big part of her life. Now, because of the risk of infection with her lymphoma and for fear of overstressing her heart, she has had to give up that pleasure. Golf — her passion over recent years — is also off the agenda, 'although the doctor would allow me to just have a little chip and putt. Can you imagine me doing only that?' she asks incredulously.

'Cancer has been a total rebirth of my life. No massages, no golf, no swimming, no running! Still, I feel no anger or bitterness. I just accept that this is my future and I have no alternative but to recognise my limitations and do my very best for myself and for my loved ones.

'Right from the beginning I never thought I was going to die — but then again, I never really dwelt on such a morbid subject. I had confidence I would get over it quickly, but I was too smart for myself and it hasn't been quick.'

Like many other women who have faced their mortality, Daphne reflects that there are always positives in any situation. 'I do think cancer has made me a better person. I am more tolerant and I am more aware of other people's problems. I can see the bigger picture of life in a clearer way. Possibly one of my best insights has been in identifying the importance of genuine friends who have wrapped me in warmth over these past years,' she says thoughtfully.

As we are finishing our chat, Daphne leans over and confides, 'I never ever thought of myself as old. Now, at 77, I am old. And I am grateful to be here, old or not. I have had a wonderful life and would not change a thing. But I am just going to stop thinking I am old!

'However, my heart grieves when I hear of the deaths of younger women who have lost the battle with this dreaded disease. They didn't even get to be old!

'I've lost two dear friends. Karen Shanks — daughter of Olympic gold medallist Norma Fleming — passed away recently after being diagnosed five years ago. Karen was my mentor during my own battle and was always there with good advice. And of course, the death of another great woman, wonderful mother and champion athlete — Kerryn McCann — was another blow,' says Daphne quietly.

Given Daphne's track record and knowing her A for Attitude outlook, I would not dismiss a comeback to international veterans' athletics in the coming years by the 'Flying Redhead' — old or not.

Hello beautiful FOAMs

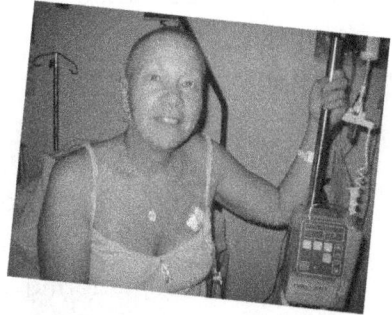

Five down only one to go! It seems to have been forever that I have juggled the three-week cycle of chemotherapy. But diary-wise it has only been almost 5 months. Let me say thank you for all your support. None of you will understand how much you have helped me through in your own individual ways — and you know how you did that.

Getting over the yukky bits. Had my fifth chemo on Monday. The gremlins were at work at the hospital that day. There weren't enough staff to do my blood test through the port so I had to go over to the blood collectors in the main hospital and have it through my saggy veins ... leaving a lovely bruise. Then after seeing my doctor (who was 40 minutes late even though I was her first appointment) I was fine to go ahead with treatment. Then my files got misplaced, so after waiting an hour I asked when I was getting chemo — and finally went in to my delivery. All went smoothly ...

But the good bit was that Pete came with me for the first time for my treatments. He knew the fifth is always a psychologically hard one and so he volunteered to be there for me. This was particularly special as Pete has an almost pathological hatred of hospitals, but he moved past that to be there for me. As he said recently on our 30th wedding anniversary, 'I'm here for the long haul — the good and the bad.' Thank you, Pete.

The hospital debacle continued, with my admission again being cancelled — no beds. Peter, doc and I made the decision to be ferried over to another private hospital, where they had a bed. Things went smoothly and I was in my bed to get through the night.

Unfortunately, for some reason I had been allocated a bed in a ward with three darling old dears — who all have severe respiratory disorders, and all spent the three days of my stay coughing and spluttering. They were quite ill, and I really felt for each of them. But as an oncology patient just having had chemotherapy, I was in a difficult position of not risking getting a respiratory infection which, as you know, is the bane of us cancer patients undergoing treatment.

When my temp started to rise up to 37.6°C late Tuesday afternoon, I felt I'd be better off at home so I discharged myself (with my doctor's permission I add, for those who worry about my independent nature).

Note to myself: If expecting to be nauseous, do NOT choose RED jelly for lunch! Very scary to nursing staff when it reappears in a kidney-shaped bowl an hour later, which prompts them to ring for help with a bleeding patient! Then the nurse realised that because the jelly had followed chemo, it is 'toxic waste', and she has to wear the total protection of gloves, glasses and coat, which caused more panic. I then had the full protective gear hung beside my bed with a note saying that it is *toxic red jelly* — not blood — for future calls.

On a completely more exciting note, I went to a very over-the-top glam ball on Friday night at the Greek Club, renowned for its big skirts and even bigger hairstyles! Oh, what to wear? And, more importantly, what to do with my bald head that has started sprouting some dark wisps on top?

Wear LBD and black veil and slink into the background? Sorry, not really me. Maybe wear elaborate bright blue wig to team with my bright blue choice of dress? Too hot when dancing and may turn green. Wrap a pearly concoction around my head with a big Indian-style drop jewel onto my forehead? Too difficult to keep in place with my energetic dancing style.

No other option than to just go bald. So silver glitter it was. I put gel onto my head and sprinkled over the silver fairy dust. Sadly, I just looked like a human disco ball!

This pondering led me to a deeper issue: Everyone keeps asking why I don't cover up. I got thinking over that — especially the words used. To me they have a connotation of something that needs to be hidden away because it is distasteful or even embarrassing, or is a bad thing — as in an attempt to hide something shameful or illegal, or make up an excuse.

My answer is always the same. At the moment this is ME. I am a woman who had breast cancer and through treatment is now bald. That is who I am. Again, God was kinder to me than I may deserve in giving me a lovely shaped head with no real bumps lumps or scars. A shame many of you won't see this new, and might I say exciting, phase in my life.

Never again will I bitch about a pimple, looking plain or a bad hair day. I will love my aged looks and my god damn happy smile. Although, God, can I pray that you just don't give me black hair with a pensioner perm look?????

Love you all

AM

Dawn Leicester's Journey

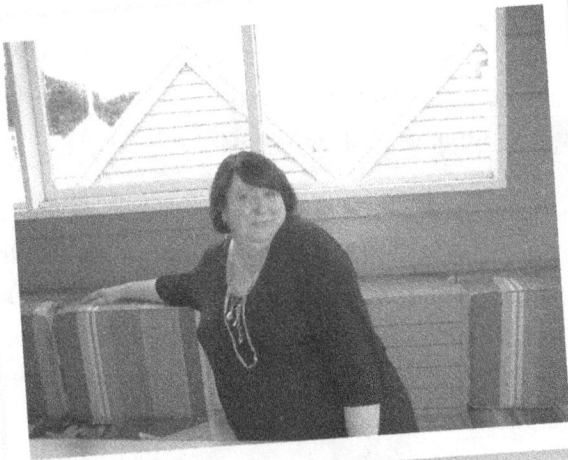

'The cancer unleashed what was always there, but I guess it gave me the courage to be genuine. I realised that I was more resilient than I thought and that was the gift this diagnosis gave me — the discovery of my own inner power.'

*D*awn Leicester and I meet in an inner-city hotel. Knowing that Dawn is probably AFL team Collingwood's number one supporter, I am not at all surprised when she walks in dressed in patriotic black and white.

As I am also a sports fan, we start a footy discussion and it is immediately obvious why Dawn wrote her popular book *Real Women Love Footy*. Dawn is a fantastic woman who is passionate about her footy. So it is ironic that at the exact time of her greatest triumph in publishing and promoting this book, Dawn also experienced her most confronting challenge when she was diagnosed with breast cancer.

'I have to say, in quoting from *A Tale of Two Cities*, for me 2003 was the best of times and the worst of times,' says Dawn. Snap! I share with her that 2003 was also when I was diagnosed with breast cancer.

On 3 September 2003, after five years of writing, planning, and finding a publisher, Dawn was celebrating the launch of her book with a big party. Her eyes twinkle as she remembers the excitement of that night. 'We had 150 of our closest friends, all of whom had to buy a book. The night was a culmination of many dreams. I had always wanted to write and, of course, I love my footy so this night was really special for me.'

At that time Dawn was a middle manager with ANZ Bank and although she lived in Melbourne she managed the bank's affairs in New South Wales. 'It was a stimulating job and I was professionally challenged and satisfied.

'When I look back, I realise what a stressful pressure-cooker environment I was living in. But at the time for me it was just a normal busy life. The added stress that my mother-in-law was in hospital for an extended period, my father-in-law had a stroke and my husband was starting a new business — plus writing the book — didn't really impact on me. In fact, I would have described my life as very exciting.'

'I had no real indication of anxiety or tension in my life — quite the opposite. I had achieved a life dream in writing the book. It seems a little silly, but when the book first came out, every time I went past a bookshop I looked at copies of my book and wanted to stroke them and the bookshelves. It was a wonderful time,' enthuses Dawn.

But, in common with many women who are diagnosed with breast cancer, she also had a niggling sense that maybe all was not so rosy. In May of that year, Dawn had what she calls 'my woman's service visit' to her doctor.

'The doctor was very efficient and said that everything looked fine, but she told me that as I had very large breasts, I should get a mammogram done in the next 12 months. There was no urgency. So I put the referral in my handbag and in all probability it would have stayed there until the next year when I saw her again.

'Then in late July, one night after I'd come home from work, I was changing into casual clothes when I scratched what I just thought was a blind pimple in my right breast. I thought nothing of it, but ten days later I noticed it was still there. I took a look and it wasn't a pimple, but there was an obvious lump.

'I knew I should get it investigated and I remembered my mammogram form. But the book launch was almost upon me, my birthday was coming up, and I decided that the screening could wait a few weeks. So I made a booking for early September,' she says.

'In hindsight I am glad I made the appointment for after the book launch as, given my diagnosis, it would have really spoiled that time. I am also very fortunate that my condition wasn't adversely affected by the three-week delay.'

Dawn had the mammogram and heard those scary words: 'There is something a little unusual and we'd like you to have an ultrasound.'

'The problem was that they couldn't give me an appointment for a whole week. There didn't seem to be any real urgency, but waiting was emotionally taxing for me,' adds Dawn.

'The first time I began to really worry was after the ultrasound when they asked me to make sure I saw my doctor that night. As it turned out, that day I was running late and rang the doctor to suggest

I reschedule. But when the receptionist told me the doctor would wait for me, I realised the news was bad,' says Dawn soberly.

'I walked in and said, "I'm crook, aren't I?" and the doctor answered, "Yes." I had two lumps and I knew I was in

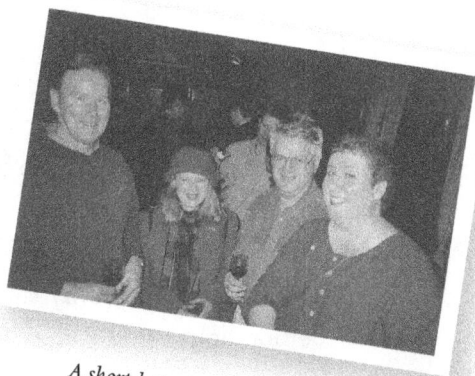

A short-haired Dawn, with friends

for a miserable six months. But I also knew that my way of dealing with things is just that — deal with them. So I just switched on to managing my cancer.'

Dawn had all the tests for secondary tumours before her surgery and so was very grateful that she knew she was only dealing with the tumours in her breast and that the cancer had not spread or metastasised.

'This was so important to know. One of my school friends had died of bone cancer in 2000 and I had nightmares about cancer being in my bones. But now I knew what I was dealing with and got on with it.'

Dawn was given the choice of a lumpectomy or the mastectomy and finally opted for a mastectomy. 'I chose to have the breast off because there were two different lumps and it was a case of "just take it away from me". If they had offered to take both breasts off, I would have done it — I just wanted it all gone,' she says decisively.

Looking back, Dawn doesn't regret having the mastectomy because she felt it was the right thing to do at the time. But she does wish she had asked more questions to understand the future impact of living with one breast.

'Later on, I made the decision that I would have a reconstruction, but before I could organise it, I had an epiphany when I was diagnosed with Type 2 diabetes. At first I was a little blasé because, after all, I had had cancer and had got through that. But my doctor made me realise that I do need to change my lifestyle and become healthy. She told me that losing weight and exercising was going to be more beneficial for me in preventing the cancer coming back than having another dose of chemotherapy. Hmm. No brain work to realise that this is the year when I am going to rebuild myself physically, and that includes having the reconstruction.'

After Dawn's mastectomy she hoped that she might be able to avoid chemotherapy or radiation. 'I thought I may avoid it by having my breast removed. But with a Grade 2 tumour and 32 nodes removed, the medical team advised me that as I was quite young — at 43, I was delighted with that! — they wanted to throw everything at me. They told me that they had looked at the pathology and as far as they could be humanly sure, I was cancer-free. However, they suggested that I have a course of chemotherapy as a precaution. Well, who would argue with that?' she asks. 'So I did it for insurance.'

The last months of 2003 were hectic ones for Dawn. As well as making critical and life-changing decisions concerning her breast cancer treatment, she was on the promotional trail, marketing her book.

'It really was frantic. I was doing radio interviews, speaking at functions and all the hoo-ha you do in publicising a book. And of course it was AFL Grand Finals time in Melbourne, and Collingwood was playing in the finals — the best time of the year! So it was probably for the best that I had to wait for a month for my surgery.

'I didn't tell most of my friends — especially my footy mates. I didn't want to ruin the fun and excitement of the Finals. It probably sounds odd, but it was much easier having cancer than telling people. I guess it was because I felt bad about making others feel bad and because I knew many thought I was going to die. It's that "You're in the coffin already" thing. I tried to find a variety of different ways to give my news to those I wanted to tell.'

She remembers telling her father by saying she was alright; but her dad immediately replied she couldn't be because she had cancer. Her mother didn't cope and took the emotional burden personally. Her footy friend Allison was caring, but with tough love she said bluntly, 'Well, you have six months to get over it, and I expect you back here ready for Round 1.'

Sadly, as experienced by many women with breast cancer, Dawn found there were friendships that will never be the same. 'They were good at the shiny bits, but couldn't cope with the darker side.'

On the positive side, her staff at ANZ were sensational. In order to distract herself, Dawn chose to continue working. Physically and emotionally it was sometimes tough. 'But I wanted to keep some normalcy in my life, and I found the love around me so empowering!

'I struggled to tell them I had cancer, so my deputy told them. But when I returned from surgery I was totally open with them and happy to talk about it. My staff really did share the experience with me; their actions spoke strongly of their support, and they kept me sane and buoyant. Their promise to me was that they would look after things at work if I promised to look after myself. We both kept our promises.'

She tells me about the day her hair started to fall out as a classic example of her relationship with her staff. 'It was a Friday afternoon in the office; I ran my fingers through my hair and I pulled out a handful. It is almost a relief because you know it is going to happen. I did it again to make sure and again hair fell out. So I rushed back to my team and told them, pulling out a handful in front of them. Then a couple of my team wanted to have a go themselves. This made a little joke of it and eased the way for me to be bald at work,' she explains with a laugh.

The next Monday, Dawn went to the hairdresser to have her head shaved and wig trimmed and turned up at work next day with what she describes as a great sexy red bob!

'I am a woman who really enjoys her hair and doing fun things with it, so losing my hair was disturbingly emotional. The wig only lasted ten days because it was summer and my scalp was hot and itchy and got infected so I thought, "Enough!" I experimented with scarves, hats and wraps. I chose lots of really bright colours and my headwear became a talking point. I wanted to remain professional but I also didn't want my baldness to stop me being stylish and looking good. It was also a great excuse to splash out on fabulous hats.' Dawn gives a laugh as she fluffs her now black stylish locks.

Whilst she acted proactively about losing her hair, Dawn was terrified that she would lose her eyebrows and eyelashes. 'When I was a little girl I had eye surgery and the doctors shaved my brows and cut my lashes. I've never forgotten that and I do admit to being a little vain about my lashes and even having a wee cry at the thought of it. I was scared I would look like a freak. Fortunately, it didn't happen.

'One of the surprising things I learned about myself, during what I would consider the potentially most unattractive months of my life, was that it became one of the most feminine experiences I have ever had. With my emphasis on my professional career, I think I had forgotten what it was like to be a girl. Focusing on my appearance boosted my morale. I've revelled in the girly things, and in the past few years I have got into perfume, wonderful clothes and being sassy.'

After laughing together about her fashion, hats, scarves, perfume and all things girly, Dawn then pauses for a few moments. She also wants to share her more serious reflections on the impact of her cancer journey.

'Cancer was probably the most important thing that has ever happened to me. I can't say I am glad it happened, because that would be a very dumb thing to say. The whole cancer experience could be destructive but instead it has given me a sense of purpose and of myself. I think it changed me as a person, unlocked my soul and shook up the real woman in me. I can be true to my authentic self. I've made sense out of cancer.

'I am stronger. I used to desperately want to please people but now I do what I want and am less apologetic about it. I say no when I want to. I remember one significant occasion about a year after my diagnosis. My close friend, Penny, who I wrote the book with, asked me to a Melbourne Football Club function. I didn't want to go so I told her I'd give it a miss. It was a real moment for me when I could say no without justifying myself. I felt liberated,' says Dawn with pride.

'The cancer unleashed what was always there, but I guess it gave me the courage to be genuine. I realised that I was more resilient than I thought and that was the gift this diagnosis gave me — the discovery of my own inner power.

'Speaking out about my journey is probably the most worthwhile thing I do now. I try to demystify cancer, to take away the fear and give people hope.

'Ironically, about three months before I got breast cancer I went to a fortune teller. She pulled out one of her cards relating to my health and told me, "You are healthy now, but within six months you will have a serious illness. Nevertheless, you will come out of it stronger than ever." At the time I went, "Right!" I'm not really a believer. However, I wonder about it now. And life isn't a rehearsal, so I am going to enjoy the life I have — now!'

Dawn is determined to savour every moment of her life. 'I don't want to be defined as Dawn Leicester, the woman who had cancer. However, I do feel I'd like to share some of my journey and maybe even impart some of the lessons I've learned during my experience. So I am writing my memoirs with a working title of *How I lost my hair and other bits*. Whether it eventually gets published is in the lap of the gods. But I loved writing the footy book and I have always wanted to be a journalist. And maybe this is cathartic for me. So I think the book fulfils what I want to do with my life at the moment.'

As the vibrant Dawn Leicester gets ready to leave, she looks me straight in the eyes and says, 'For both of us, 2003 was a dreadful year — getting breast cancer. But for me, the greatest tragedy of that year was that Collingwood lost the Grand Final — and to your team!'

This real woman really loves her footy!

For the record:

BRISBANE LIONS: 5.5, 11.7, 14.12, **20.14 (134)**

COLLINGWOOD: 3.3, 4.7, 9.7, **12.12 (84)**

Hello everyone

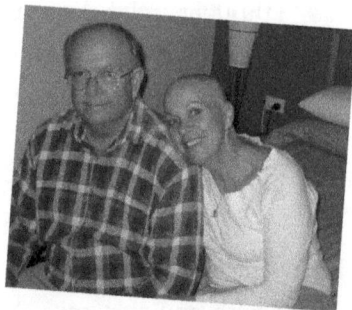

Thought I would share my *Bald and Bootiful* look with those of you whom I haven't seen for a while ... would hate you to walk past me in the street 'cos you didn't recognise me.

Vanesa has already warned me not to wear my leather pants in case people are scared of the smiling skinhead — and that's without the dog collar and nose ring!

Please note how perfectly I can now draw on eyebrows and thicken up the 16 eyelashes I still have!

And you can see that Peter is covering his excitement at being forced to smile for the paparazzi!!

AM

Margaret Stewart's Journey

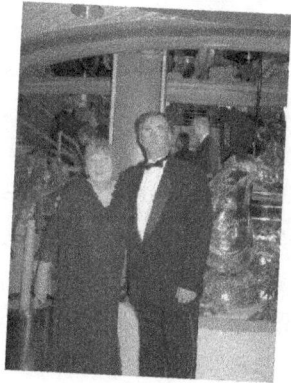

'If there is a positive to be taken from this story, then it is that the publicity surrounding the possible cancer cluster has attracted a lot of attention from researchers ... some research is fast-tracked and maybe, just maybe, the doctors will find ... that elusive cure for breast cancer.'

Margaret Stewart is a self-confessed loud and gregarious mother hen. But behind her extroverted nature lies a deeply compassionate and humble woman with the proverbial heart of gold.

We sit talking on her deck as Queensland media news outlets tell of the Australian Broadcasting Corporation's plan to relocate their new Queensland studios to South Bank Parklands in central Brisbane. This corporate move is one of the epilogues in Margaret's story. Margaret has worked at the ABC Television studios in Brisbane for over 20 years part-time as a News Operator Assistant — a job she loves doing and with a 'great group of mates and work colleagues'.

She was diagnosed in 2004 with breast cancer, but her journey begins several years earlier. 'Before I was diagnosed, I did know a little about breast cancer because a few of the girls at the ABC had been diagnosed with the disease. I was also fairly aware of breast cancer because of the publicity and promotion that surrounds mammogram testing and self-examination. In fact, I had been having mammograms myself for several years and I was quite vigilant in making my friends get tested. I've even been known to make appointments for them and make them keep them.

'When one of the girls in my news area was diagnosed in the 1990s, it did make me personally more aware of the effects of being diagnosed. That woman was a very private person and so I hadn't realised in the beginning that it was breast cancer. I think our group of workmates were there for her, but I don't think she realised we were. In hindsight, she needed our support and the support of management, but one must respect another's privacy.

'Then another woman was diagnosed. She was more outgoing, and people asked after her and looked out for her. She later decided to leave the ABC and we all wished her well.

'So even with a couple of cases close to me, I never thought there was any real significance to what was happening and I just saw it as a bit of a coincidence. We had quite a lot of women working in the news room and so I just thought it was chance and bad luck that some women had been diagnosed with breast cancer,' admits Margaret.

'Then, in 2001, my good friend in news production gave me the bad news that she, too, had breast cancer. I was devastated. I remember going out and meeting her for a coffee in her suburb and reassuring her I'd be there for her, and she'd be fine. I was just shattered at her diagnosis. But, again, I didn't see it for more than that my friend was bloody unlucky.'

At around the same time, Margaret had her own scare.

'My family were due to go away on holidays, and I was visiting my one-in-a-million GP. I'd had a mammogram late in October 2000 but as we were heading overseas, he said he'd better do a thorough check-up. He then found a lump.

'I remember ringing work and telling them I would be a little bit late as my doctor had found a lump in my breast and I had to get it checked out as soon as possible. On the other end of the line my workmate said, "Gee, you're funny. You really crack a good joke." I told her I was not joking, and when I sobbed on the phone she realised it wasn't a joke. This was very serious and I was off to have an ultrasound.

Margaret was very relieved when she received the news that the lump was benign.

'In the next few years, there were a few more cases of breast cancer at work — although the women who were diagnosed worked in different sections. In 2002 a journalist was diagnosed, and some of the staff became a little concerned and were rallying around investigating and creating files on potential radiation risks and other possible causes. But I just thought it was a series of coincidences. I knew the fact that one in 11 women in Australia is diagnosed with breast cancer and I guess I just thought our group at work was a bit unlucky,' says Margaret.

'I appreciated what the people at work were doing but I didn't know enough about the facts. Truly, I still just thought it was darn bad luck that we were seeing women regularly being diagnosed with breast cancer at our workplace. But with the new diagnoses, people were looking back at these increasing numbers. And with hindsight they were sensing there were more women diagnosed than was normal and they were wondering why.'

Although several people in her department were researching breast cancer and looking for answers and explanations on the internet, and making notes and circulating ideas and causes, Margaret did not become involved in this. 'I had — and still do have — enormous respect for my colleagues, but all the information was complicated and a bit above me and I kept believing that it was just coincidence.'

Because of the suspicious lump that had been found in her breast earlier, Margaret was scheduled for mammograms and ultrasounds every six months. In 2004, after one of her regular check-ups, the radiologist picked up a suspicious collection of cells and suggested she follow it through with her specialist, who then said she had to have a needle biopsy.

'My daughter came with me to the hospital to have this procedure and I was a little concerned that things weren't too good — you'd be silly if you didn't worry when you'd been asked to have a biopsy, wouldn't you? I was supposed to go back for the results, but instead, being a casual sort of person, I asked for the results over the phone to save me having to drive out to the surgery. They told me I had to make an appointment to come in to talk to the doctor and get the results. So I made that appointment prior to my going to work.

'When I sat down, the doctor gave me the bad news that I had cancer: ductal carcinoma in situ. I was by myself and I was in shock. I didn't take in a single word he said. It hit me then. I know he was talking about cancer, and telling me things that I needed to know, but I was away with the fairies,' she says.

'In fact, I had heard nothing after the C word and so I had to ring him back the next day to ask for information. He then explained everything to me again and gave me a concise picture of what I needed to do. So at least then I knew what I was in for.

'After being told I had breast cancer, I went back to work. I remember my mate in production looking at me as I came in. She knew I'd been for tests and when I looked at her, she knew it was bad.

Immediately, I hurried out of the room. I was very emotional. I was advised to go home, but me being me, I said, "No, I'll stay," and I even asked one of my team to go over the road and buy a cake. Cakes solve everything!'

Indeed, Margaret is famous for her caramel tarts and patty cakes. 'I guess I am the mum figure at work, and cakes brighten us up, so it was just a normal response when there was a tense situation to "feed the team cake,"' she jokes.

'I then came back into the office and heard everyone muttering and wondering. So I stood up in front of them all and said, "We are a news room and I have had some bad new today. And, yes, it is breast cancer. So now you know, let's get on with work."'

Margaret then rang her husband, Al, and told him the bad news. 'When my daughter, Amanda, rang me, she asked me how I got on, and I told her I didn't have A, didn't have B, but had C. Then my son, Michael, rang a little later and I could tell he didn't know what to say.

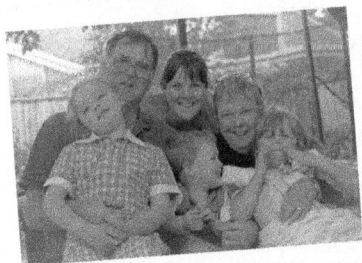

Margaret with her husband, daughter and grandchildren

'I actually had found it very hard to tell Al and the kids. It's really tough on the family. No one knows what to say. I truly believe that those around us are more affected by our diagnosis than we are ourselves,' Margaret explains. 'They often feel that they are powerless to help.

'When I had spoken to Al straight after I got my results, I asked him to get together with Michael and Amanda and I would see them all later. So he and the kids had a family conference before I got home from work that night. That meant that, even though they were all very emotional, they had talked things through and were ready and prepared to help me.

'Fortunately, I didn't have to go through chemotherapy, but I did have the full gamut of radiation sessions. I kept working all through my treatments. I'd go up to the hospital and have the last appointment on the radiation machine each night.'

Meanwhile, back at the ABC studios, after Margaret's diagnosis suspicions started to get stronger that perhaps there was a problem. 'Three of us who sat at the same desk had now got breast cancer, as well as others in the news room. I remember one journalist who now sat next to me saying that she hoped it wasn't contagious. I said to her, "It's breast cancer not bloody diarrhoea," and laughed.

'And would you believe it — just a few weeks later that woman didn't appear at work. I asked where she was and no one knew why she wasn't working. After a week I rang her at home and asked her if she was okay. Two days later I read a general staff email telling us that this woman had just been diagnosed with breast cancer.'

'I must admit, that afternoon I lost the plot. That young woman sat beside me at the same production desk, so that was one more diagnosis. Cancer is so scary. I was becoming a little concerned. This woman was young, beautiful and had young children. Life wasn't fair that she should cop this. I felt very guilty that I had a good diagnosis and she seemed to have a tough one,' says Margaret.

'This new cancer identification seemed to be the catalyst for an increase in suspicions about the unusually large number of breast cancer diagnoses at the Toowong studios of the ABC. I went to the boss and said that I thought the ABC needed to be more sensitive in dealing with us and asked that they communicate in a more open manner.

'And from then, I do believe that the majority of management began to take notice of our concerns,' she says.

Things settled a little at the ABC office, with no new diagnoses for about a year. Margaret had just finished her treatment and was back to getting on with her life. 'I'd come back to work after Christmas and one of my good friends at work hadn't come back from holidays and I knew she was due back. So in late January I rang her and was a bit cheeky saying, "Where the heck are you?"

'My friend told me she couldn't talk to me. I persisted, saying, "Hold on, this is your surrogate mum here," and she still wouldn't tell me anything. That worried me. This young woman is like a daughter to me, and my heart started pumping because I knew something wasn't right. Finally, she told me she, too, had breast cancer. I just couldn't believe it,' says Margaret. The pain of that memory is still raw, and tears start spilling down her cheeks.

'I remember phoning my close friend at work and relaying the news to her. She was so distraught that I phoned the boss to say I was concerned about her driving to work. She was very angry and upset. She told her superior that something had to be done as this wasn't right.

'My friend had a really rough time with cancer. And it was yet another young one from work — and she'd just had her first mammogram. I am close to her and her family. I felt once again devastated. But I hope we were there for her and helped in some small way.

'I remember her having to have a serious test; her work colleagues knew about this. I said, "Look, I don't care if you are Catholic, Protestant, Anglican or an unbeliever — just get out of bed tomorrow and say a prayer to someone that this test goes well." We would know the results at 5.30 that afternoon. It was really great to see everyone just beaming at the news that the test was clear; we were just relieved and so overjoyed. There is no point crying in front of these young people; you need to be strong and listen to them and then go away and cry. But I do feel for them — I guess I am just a mother hen.

'It was only then — after that girl's diagnosis — that I began thinking that maybe there was something going on at the studios. She also sat at that same production desk, so I finally acknowledged that maybe it was a little more than a coincidence,' recalls Margaret.

'I did respect the opinions of my colleagues who believed there was a serious problem and that a cancer cluster was forming. I have always been very supportive of other people and their thoughts and ideas and continued to listen to what they had to say, even though I'd argue with them. Morale was very low, and I was starting to change my thinking.

'But my real issue was not why this was happening; for me, it was that I continued to feel guilty. I was the oldest person diagnosed, and my diagnosis was not as serious as the other women, and they were all so young. I almost felt a little bit of a fraud.

'Funnily enough, when I was diagnosed I never asked, "Why me?" I never felt sorry for myself, because there were always people around me who were far worse off.'

This new diagnosis was also a call to action for ABC Management. Several journalists were very vocal about the need to scrutinise the situation and protect the staff. The ABC brought in a psychologist and a doctor to work with the staff, and employed a radiation investigator. A full staff meeting was also organised to discuss the state of affairs.

'At that meeting, one of the young reporters stood up and said very vehemently that she thought every woman in the ABC should have a mammogram and an ultrasound because there had been just too many cases here. That girl was so concerned that she had already rung up to make an appointment for a mammogram. She'd been told she was young and fit and didn't need one. But she insisted that the doctors give her one for her own peace of mind. She just needed to know that she was safe,' explains Margaret.

'Just a few days later she rang me to tell me something I just did not want to hear. She had breast cancer. Again, I was totally devastated. It was extremely distressing — and again, she sat at the same desk. That girl finally left the ABC and journalism to pursue a new life. Although I don't see her here at work, she is always in my thoughts.'

Around the same time as the latest upheavals at the ABC, Margaret's daughter's young friend died of breast cancer. Margaret felt almost overcome by the devastation that breast cancer was wreaking around her.

'I couldn't help thinking, "Why the young?" That's when the horrendous nature of this disease hit home, and when that happened I just thought how lucky I was. I am trying to live now and not worry about what may happen in the future.

'Living positively was always going to be easier said than done. During this time, I was told that my daughter and family were moving interstate with the grandchildren and also my close neighbour was moving to the country. I didn't accept this news well. In fact, one could say I stuffed up. I probably ruined a great relationship that will most likely never be the same. I was advised to get psychiatric help to deal with all the goings-on and had a great doctor. But even to this day I have trouble dealing with the family separation, even though I realise they must lead their own lives. I just miss them dearly.

'Things at work were getting very grim, and when we had yet another case, I don't think it is exaggerating to say that all of the young women at work were now looking around and wondering who would be next. Personally, it was overwhelming for me to see these young women being almost picked off, one after the other. I admit to becoming very emotional at this time.'

This newest case was the catalyst for many of the staff at the ABC studios at Toowong to decide enough was enough and they staged a very public walkout.

'I joined the staff in leaving the studios. Being an oldie, I was wondering about causes, but I still tried to keep an open mind. I kept thinking about the high statistical rate of women getting breast cancer, but logic told me that there certainly did seem to be a level of abnormality at the ABC.

'The last diagnosis before we left Toowong was the last straw. I could see the staff was very troubled. A news room deals on a daily basis with death, trauma and unpleasant realities, and I accept that we may become a little immune to shock, although at times we would shed tears at sad news. We're not heartless. But when it's close to you — people at the same desk; friends, colleagues and workmates — it is a totally different kettle of fish.'

A delegate came from Sydney to talk with the staff, who then voted to move out of the Toowong studios. 'I knew this was a big resolution because it meant shifting the whole organisation. This would affect the lives of so many people who worked here. So this was a huge decision,' says Margaret.

'We then had a new Managing Director, Mark Scott, who was quick off the mark to try to settle the anxiety. He listened to us and was sympathetic to what was happening to the women. He engaged

Professor Armstrong, a renowned Director of Research at the NSW Cancer Council, to do a scientific investigation to find a possible cause for the elevated occurrence of breast cancer here at Toowong.

'Mark Scott has always been there to listen to our concerns. This is how he was to me. Even though others in the ABC may have their own views, this is how I see it. These people were tremendous.

'We were due to have a meeting with Mark Scott, and the old saying, "It doesn't rain but it pours," rang true. My husband — who is such a support and a great guy — said, "I know it's not a very convenient time but I think I've had a stroke." Believe it or not, we had a laugh about it and proceeded straight to the hospital, where he spent three weeks. We are so lucky he got back the use of the parts affected by the stroke and is doing well now.

'Then a day or two before Christmas 2006, all the staff was called in for a meeting at 10am. I wasn't starting work until mid-afternoon and I was in the middle of my mad Christmas preparation rush. So I wasn't a happy camper. I retorted that I would come in but that they needed to put aside a car park for a "mentally challenged mad Marg"! But I knew it was important to be there.

'Professor Armstrong's interim report was being handed down. Everyone was very shocked that it was his recommendation that the ABC needed to move its site. After telling us his recommendations, we were instructed to go to our own supervisors and then we were advised that we would be leaving the building in ten minutes.

'I was very sad and I couldn't believe that I was leaving the building and workplace I'd been working in for so many years. My life, and those of all of us at the ABC, was changed for ever. We were being split into about nine different worksites around Brisbane, so this was a major decision to relocate the ABC. The whole breast cancer story affected a greater number of people than you would realise.

'Since the upheaval, many people lost the jobs they used to do, and in some cases their positions were no longer in existence. We are working in challenging conditions. But the staff at ABC is very resilient and I think their caring, their camaraderie and great sense of humour has seen us through very, very tough times. I look on them as part of my family.

'If there is a positive to be taken from this story, then it is that the publicity surrounding the possible cancer cluster has attracted a lot of attention from researchers, who are searching for answers. I am positive that the high profile our group has achieved meant that some research is fast-tracked and maybe, just maybe, the doctors will find answers for us and hopefully that elusive cure for breast cancer,' says Margaret optimistically.

'I have no bitterness about my diagnosis or my employer and I look forward to seeing the results of all the research that has evolved out of our workplace at the ABC. Professor Armstrong's final report proved there was no radiation. So I am still open-minded about causes — even though there have been several more diagnoses revealed in the last year or so.'

The final report also excluded all other environmental causes for the high incidence of cancer, and was unable to identify any reason for the increase in risk.

'My focus was never on blame or fault. It is just devastatingly unfair that the young ones at work were given such a tough road,' she says.

'It's a difficult thing to say, but I guess I actually wanted the worst diagnosis for me and an easier one for those with long lives ahead of them. That guilt has badly affected me and I still carry sadness about that. I'm not a saint or a martyr or stupid; it is just that my heart goes out to all of those workmates having to go through breast cancer.'

I am sure that all of those women at the ABC who did go through their breast cancer journey are grateful that Mad Marg — with her cakes, her love and her caring generosity — was there to look after them and make their journey just that much easier to travel.

The names of women diagnosed with breast cancer at the ABC have been omitted to protect their privacy.

Hello lovely FOAMs

Thought I'd share two pieces of good news.

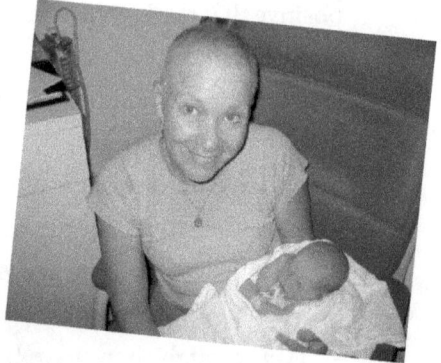

The first is the birth of my beautiful second granddaughter, Ella Grace, who was born at 2.02am Thursday September 25th. She is so gorgeous and at only 28 hours old she has more hair than me. She is the most beautiful little human soul and only one of the amazing reasons to be grateful for being wonderfully alive. Ben and Kylie and little Madeleine Kate are so thrilled to welcome Ella to their family. It is also a reminder that family is always the most wonderful and important thing in life ... to be treasured.

The second piece of good news is that I have my FINAL chemo on Monday. This is the start of my physical recovery, and although I have until the middle of December with radiotherapy, the end of chemo signals the return to great health for me. In order to ensure I give myself the best opportunity to be fit and healthy I have taken a week off work and intend to nurture myself.

Enjoy the pic of Ella Grace.

AM

Khim Ung's Journey

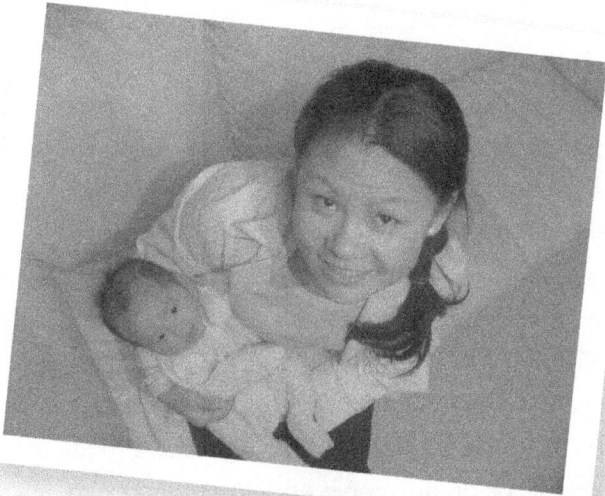

*'My early experiences ... mean that I do understand poverty ...
I realised that I wanted to go back to the place of my birth
and do something to help the country. I knew that having also
survived breast cancer at a young age, I could try to use my
saved life to make a difference.'*

As I chat to the sparkly Khim Ung, she is holding her daughter, Lillian, born just five days earlier. Little Lillian is a precious gift that Khim had not expected would ever arrive, but the doting first-time mum is revelling in the joys and pride of parenthood.

Khim laughs easily. However, her infectious personality belies the steely determination and courage that has seen her escape the Khmer Rouge, battle with breast cancer and then give back to her homeland in an extraordinary act of altruism.

Because she feared it may never happen, motherhood is now her focus, and somehow the challenges that have beset her over the past few years fade away.

'When I was diagnosed with breast cancer, I was told by my specialist that there would be a high probability that the chemotherapy would destroy my chances of having children in the future. But here I am, nearly four years later, cuddling my beautiful little girl,' says Khim.

'And adding to that miracle, Lillian was conceived naturally too! Talk about miracles on top of miracles!

'When I finished my treatments, my husband and I worried about whether we should attempt pregnancy. We agonised over whether trying to have a child was the right thing to do. My form of breast cancer feeds on hormones and, as you know, there's nothing like pregnancy for sending a woman's hormones into overdrive!' explains Khim.

'Sometimes, while I was expecting, I worried that even though I was confident that I have treated my cancer successfully, there may be tiny cancer cells still lurking somewhere in my body. I knew that if there were cells in my body, that they were non-threatening at that moment. But I was still very concerned. Could my pregnancy wake them up? The answer is, "Nobody really knows."

'But we decided that we would like a family and were thrilled when I fell pregnant. The baby and I were healthy all through my pregnancy. And now look at Lillian,' Khim says, her face beaming.

'In life we have to make decisions that others may feel are foolish, or even consider are really crazy risks. I know there was a chance that if the cancer came back that I would be leaving my daughter without a mother at a young age.

'But the decision was one I made with conviction. I decided to choose faith — faith in my body, faith in my instincts and confidence in my future. Anyone who has ever had breast cancer — or any kind of cancer — knows that faith can often seem lost when faced with this disease.

'Having this baby means that I've got my life back. When she came into the world, it was my promise to her and my husband that I intend to be here for a long, long time,' Khim says. And there can be no doubting the aura of strength around this petite, dark-haired young woman.

Research in Australia shows that in any one year about 345 people *under* the age of 40 are diagnosed with breast cancer. For any young person, such a diagnosis is very confronting, but for Khim Ung the news came at what should have been a blissful time of her life — she found her tumour almost immediately after her wedding.

'Just one month after my honeymoon, I felt a small hard lump on my right breast. The thing was, I wasn't worried because I was very young. Like many young people, I thought to myself that breast cancer is an older women's disease. So there was no way that I could imagine that this little lump would be something as serious as breast cancer,' says Khim

'But I was so wrong. In 2005, I was diagnosed with breast cancer at the age of 27 years. This was, of course, devastating. I was just married, I had my whole life ahead of me — and here I was facing cancer.'

'The cancer was worse than the doctors and I initially thought. Because my tumour was positioned so close to my lymph nodes, it meant I had an increased risk — they told me as much as a 30 per cent — that the cancer may have spread through the lymphatic system to the rest of my body. So, three years shy of my 30th birthday I immediately had a lumpectomy and had some lymph nodes removed.

'Like most people with breast cancer, I then went through the long, hard, soul-destroying months of treatment — chemotherapy, radiation therapy and hormone therapy. My body and my mind felt totally wrecked and it took every ounce of strength just to get up in the morning.

'But I know I am blessed in many ways. Imagine if I was not in Australia but back in my home country, Cambodia, a Third World country? What would my treatment have been like there? Imagine if I hadn't felt the lump so early and had surgery and all the medical care so quickly? I am so lucky; it could be much worse,' she says.

Khim tells me that only days ago, she had been speaking with a friend of hers who has just turned 60 and had been diagnosed with cancer two years earlier.

'He went through his battles and he has inspired me and influenced a lot of my ideas and attitudes. I remember one day he said to me he felt lucky that he didn't have cancer when he was young. I remember replying to him that I don't feel lucky being given breast cancer at this age but I don't feel sorry for myself either. I think there's a gift in each suffering and the gift that I got from having gone through breast cancer is that I learned my lessons at a young age.

'By having to go through all of the treatments, I learned a new kind of personal courage and I started to refocus my life. For the first time I really started putting myself first and I did things that I wanted to do,' explains Khim

'I learned that life *is* too short to do things I didn't want to do. I learned that it's *okay* to be different. I learned that it is important to do things *now*. And, most importantly, I learned that life *is* uncertain, so why wait! So, of course, I eat dessert first now,' she laughs.

After her treatments were finished, Khim, who is a designer, took a year off and worked part-time.

'But I realised something was missing in my life. I was certainly glad to have come through the cancer, but I was looking for something meaningful to make my life worthwhile at the deepest level.'

Being diagnosed with breast cancer made Khim realise the importance of her heritage and her cultural past. Khim was born in Cambodia during the Pol Pot era.

'My parents, with my one-year-old sister and I, fled Cambodia — twice. The first time, we were caught by the Thai soldiers and thrown in jail. The second time, the soldiers were so drunk during the Thai New Year that we managed to run across the border into the Red Cross Refugee Camp at Khao-I-Dang,' recalls Khim.

Khim, who was only a toddler at the time, doesn't remember much about the Cambodian war but she says that the stories her parents told her inspire her to find inner strength during difficult times. She then relates the most extraordinary tale of courage and faith, saying she believes that the fact that she is alive today is undeniably due to a series of amazing circumstances she can only call her miracles.

'The war with the Khmer Rouge started in 1975. My mother was pregnant with me in the midst of chaos. My dad was sent to work in a different province and only came home every six months. Mum was sent to work every day on the rice fields from 6am to 9pm, with just one meal to sustain her and her pregnancy. She suffered from malnutrition, her body so bloated that she was bedridden for the entire third trimester. There were no doctors, nor any medicine to cure her. She was sent home from the hospital to die with me inside her. Two days before Chinese New Year, the first miracle happened: she gave birth to me. I was only 2 kilograms in weight.

'Then, after just three weeks, the Khmer Rouge sent Mum back to work at the rice farm. I was placed in "childcare" with 50 other children. Every evening, after 10pm, Mum would pick me up and take me home. One day she noticed that the babies were slowly dying from dysentery, which had broken out among them. Mum, who previously was a nurse, knew she had to do something quickly. Secretly, she swapped her watch — the only thing of value she had — for medicine. Every night, she would secretly inject me with the medicine. By week two, almost every child had died. I was one of the very few that lived. Mum risked her life to save me. If she had been caught, she would have been executed. This was the second miracle.

'The third miracle was the first time we attempted to escape Cambodia to Thailand. At the time, Mum was pregnant with my younger sister and I was a toddler sitting on Dad's shoulders. We had nothing, no money or gold; nothing except for the clothes on our back. My parents knew it was a risky decision — it was a choice between starving in Cambodia or risking our lives for the unknown. If we were caught by the Thai soldiers, it could mean death. There were rumours that when the refugees were caught, the Thai soldiers sent them into the mountains, where death was almost a certainty. The mountains were filled with mines set by the Khmer Rouge.

'As soon as we ran across the gate, the Thai soldiers started shooting at us. We held up our hands and were dragged into jail. The cell was cold and dark. Dad begged for a blanket for Mum. One of the soldiers pitied Mum and threw in a dusty rice sack and Dad quickly ripped the sack open to cover Mum's pregnant body. Astonishingly, they saw something shiny. Sewn on the inside edge of the bag was a gold necklace with a beautiful jade pendant. Our third miracle! With half of the gold necklace, we were able to bribe the soldiers to send us back to Cambodia rather than into the mountains, and the other half bought us food and goods to sustain ourselves until the next escape into Thailand,' Khim says.

'The miracles that we encountered make me think I must have been saved for a reason. Knowing that gives me meaning to my life and strength to live every day.'

In 1983, five-year-old Khim and her family migrated to Australia, and although her refugee family was poor, life in her new country was safe, and here she had a future.

'When we came to Australia, we had nothing. Furniture, clothes, cutlery were all donated by the Salvation Army. We stayed at a friend's place for a while until we had enough money to rent a single bedroom flat. My parents worked weekdays and weeknights and weekends and they tried to save money in almost everything. There were no day outings, movies; no toys or clothes. Sometimes money was so tight that Dad had to buy live chickens to kill and cook because it was cheaper than the chicken in the supermarket,' she remembers.

'My early experiences and those of my family mean that I do understand poverty and what it means to live without food and medicine. I realised that I wanted to go back to the place of my birth and do something to help the country. I knew that having also survived breast cancer at a young age, I could try to use my saved life to make a difference.' Khim says these words with a humility and directness that would soften the most hardened cynic.

Through the Australian Youth Ambassador program, Khim decided to go to Cambodia and work in an orphanage. 'Being a part of the AYA program meant that financially I was able to afford to take time off and work in Cambodia. Cancer had given me a deeper insight and appreciation of the gift of my life. I knew that this was something I needed to do for myself but also something that would benefit the children of Cambodia.

'My husband was a little sceptical at first, but I was very determined to do this journey. I knew that this was just something I had to do — and that I would do it by myself if necessary. Fortunately, my husband understood the intenseness of my desire to go back and help my country, and he came with me.

'The desperate poverty was overwhelming. I worked with 45 children between four and 14 years of age, helping to develop health and educational programs that would make their lives just that little bit easier. I wanted to give these children a chance to live a happy, healthy and fulfilling life. It was the despair, the hopelessness of the plight of the children, that gave me hope. It made me feel I was contributing, and that was very satisfying,' adds Khim.

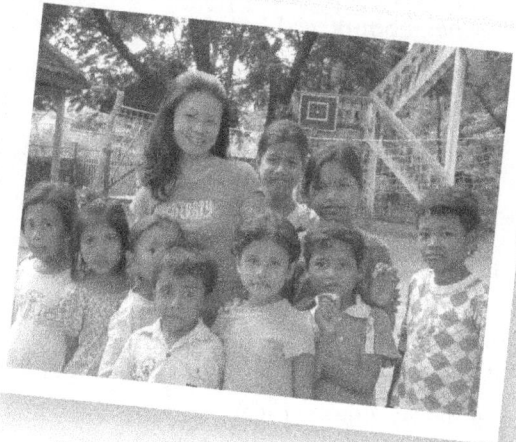

Khim surrounded by Cambodian orphans

'No matter what happens in my life, I'm sure that I will never forget my first experience of bringing a new child from her village into the orphanage. One of our staff was told about a little girl by the chief of the village. She was 11 years old and both her parents had recently died of HIV while working in Thailand. She was living with her sick and poor grandmother. To survive, they both ate leftovers from their relatives.

'The road to her village was very hot, dusty and bumpy. On the way there, we passed farmers working in rice paddocks, children walking to school and women shopping at the market. When we arrived, I saw a skinny girl in ragged clothes, running towards her fragile grandmother, who was sitting on the wooden slats outside her home. Like most poor children, she looked much younger than her 11 years. When we met, she introduced herself by raising both her hands in a prayer-like manner, head bowed. "*Chum reap sure* [Hello]," she greeted us. We joined her grandmother and we all sat down. We spoke about everything — why we were here, how we could help them, their difficulties and their hopes. They told us about her parents and her 15-year-old brother, who had left two years ago and they don't know where he is. I could see in their eyes that the pain was still very raw.

'During our conversation, I noticed that over 20 of their neighbours had surrounded us, curious and interested as to why we were there. They listened attentively. Her grandmother told us that she could no longer feed both of them nor send her grandchild to school. She then conceded that if her grandchild went to the orphanage, at least she only needed to worry about herself. "I am going to die soon but now I can rest knowing that she is being looked after," she said.

'This little girl came to me holding a bag of her belongings. Inside were an old school uniform and an old exercise book. She told me she enjoyed school and all she wanted was to learn. Through her tears she said, "Grandmother, uncles, aunties and friends, I am going now." One shouted, "You come back and visit, you hear?" Another relative added, "Don't you forget us." Her grandmother finally said, "Be a good girl," and she shoved all the money she had into her granddaughter's small hand.

'This experience will always remain with me — to see and to feel how desperate people can be. Now I can truly say that I understand the value of orphanages in Cambodia. They are not just a home for vulnerable children but a place of hope for a better future.

'By going back to Cambodia and seeing the plight of the helpless children, seeing the desperate poverty, I had a much clearer understanding of who I am, where I came from and what my parents went through during the war. It helped me to become a stronger person.

'We had planned to go for just the one year, but we stayed for six further months and only decided to come home when we found I was pregnant. We wanted to share the wonderful experience of parenthood with family and friends. We also wanted to protect this new life back home in Australia.

'Both my husband and I enjoyed living and working in Cambodia. It was certainly a life-changing experience. That chapter is now closed but another has just opened — motherhood,' Khim says, her face wreathed in smiles as she cradles her precious daughter.

'For now I just want to live simply. And maybe one day, another miracle will happen and Lillian can have a brother or sister.'

I see in Khim Ung a woman with a deep appreciation of all the goodness in her life. By delivering a healthy baby after licking cancer, she has defied the odds. In fact, I will always associate her with miracles. Her birth was a miracle — and so was her own daughter's — and she has worked hard to bring about miraculous change in the lives of others.

Well, beautiful FOAMs, I have finally finished my chemotherapy. And it is only now that I can really admit that there were times when I could only dream of this day.

It wasn't that my chemotherapy was so difficult: I know there would have been many people who had much tougher times. Not that it took so long: because 5 months in the big scheme of my wonderful life isn't that long. And it wasn't even that I suffered all that much: it was unpleasant and pesky, but not true suffering like many others may have experienced.

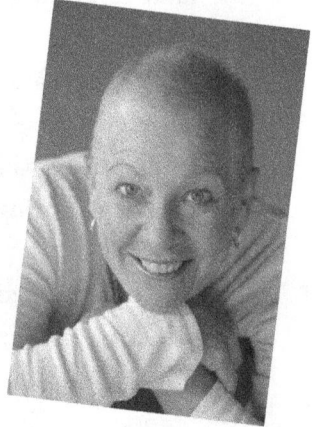

No, the real joy of finishing is that I now have some feeling of myself back. The chemotherapy dominated my life so much over the past 5 months that I never felt I was really me.

My life was divided into three AnneMaries: *chemo week*, which meant hospital for three days, vomiting, nausea and tiredness and a generally weakened disposition. Then came *nearly there but not quite week*, when I could start to eat and keep food in, I could go on slow morning walks, but the bone marrow needle supplement meant my bones and joints ached and I had flu symptoms. Finally my *good week* arrived and I could drink and eat (fortunately, the mouth ulcers haven't come back recently) and I could run, do weights and climb the steps and even stay up after the News at night!!!

From October 2003 onwards I can be AnneMarie again. And I so look forward to now living all those dreams I have, of playing again with all you wonderful people, of being able to spend time with Pete, Vanesa, Ben and his gorgeous girls, Kylie, Maddie and Ella, of being fit and healthy and sporty again. And, most of all, thinking about the exciting future that beckons ... not the next treatment!

Most importantly of all at this time, I want to give heartfelt thanks to all of you for your wonderful support. I am truly humbled and blessed that you all have, in your uniquely individual ways, made me feel loved and cared for. I have two recurring thoughts about the support of the Fab FOAMs:

The first is the story of 'Footprints'. You know the one? Where the man who is dying looks back over his life and says to God that he felt let down by God. He told God that God had promised to walk with him in his life, but as he looked back at the footprints in the sands of his life, he noticed during the difficult times there was only one pair of footprints. 'Why, God, did you abandon me?' he asked. 'I did not abandon you. Rather, during the difficult times, I carried you, and that's why there is only one set of footprints.'

So many of you helped me at times when I felt I was trudging uphill on a sandy mountain. It may have been a hug or cuddle, phone call, a note, an SMS text or an email, home-cooked meals, a visit with muffins or rich chocolates, a scarf to knit, flowers after each chemo, massages, offers to stay or host a lunch for me, even a lucky fairy garden to wish in.

Things that may have seemed insignificant to you, but came at just the moment for me — when I need a lift.

The other thought is of Mark Twain's book and the Mike and the Mechanics song. I feel like Huckleberry Finn and Tom Sawyer — attending their own funeral in their LIVING YEARS. I have had but a glimpse of people's care and affection during my journey thus far with breast cancer. Mostly we have to wait until we die to know that people actually really cared about us. How blessed am I to have been given this special gift in my 'living years'. Thank you, dear friends.

I now have a three-week recovery period and then have radiation treatment each day from the end of October until mid-December. However, it is not as intrusive as chemo, and although it creates tiredness, I am told by others it is a breeze compared to chemo.

By Christmas I will be celebrating like an angel and my New Year's resolution will be a simple thank you for the past and being able to give back in the future! Every day for me has always been a special moment to enjoy. Now I know the truth of this, I intend to not only enjoy each day for the rest of my long and disgraceful life, but to be truly grateful!!!

Thank you again FAB FOAMs for getting me through chemo ...

Smile

AM

Anni Franklin Wood's Journey

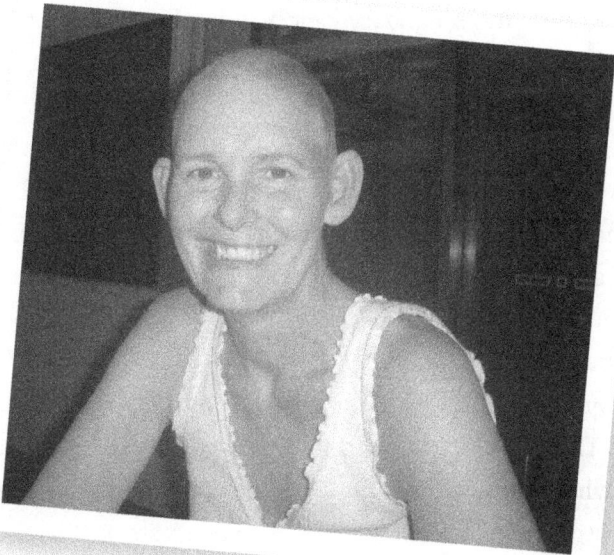

'I'd got to a stage that I felt I was always complaining about insignificant things, that I was being neurotic and imagining pains and problems. I felt I was becoming a hypochondriac so I said nothing. Now I tell everyone whenever I can, "If you have any pain, no matter how slight, you go to the doctor."'

When Anni and I first met, we were posing for a promotional photo for the Pink Ribbon Breakfasts with international swimming legend Susie O'Neill. The photo shoot was happening poolside and our information brief said *swimsuits and T-shirts*. To say we were both feeling a little daunted was an understatement.

Changing into our pink T-shirts covering our togs, we simultaneously looked at each other and laughed as Anni said: 'What are we worried about — we're alive!'

That positive energy and optimistic attitude still shine out of her, even though she admits to being frail, weak and struggling with her health. Anni has secondary cancer in her bones, liver, breast and brain and even simple tasks like walking and driving a car are now challenges — but don't tell this powerhouse that!

When I arrive at Anni's home to do the interview for this book, I receive a warm welcome. Family photos dot the wall, and I can see that Anni is a person who surrounds herself with love. A passionate woman, she insists, 'I'm not done yet! Oh no, this isn't going to get me — yet. I think that approach is important. Sadly some people do give up, but I won't.

'When I wake up I look at the photo of my daughter, Laura, beside my bed. That is reason enough to get out of bed ready for another day; it's what keeps me battling on. And every morning my husband, Mark, brings me my morning tea in bed and treats me like a princess. He is my partner in all of this and gives me the encouragement and strength I need at times. I'd be lost without him.'

In 2000 Anni was a federal public servant living an everyday normal life in Canberra with her husband and young daughter. 'Life was good but I really hated the cold. So after 11 years in Canberra and with Laura ready to start school, it seemed like the perfect time for our family to move north.'

Anni arrived in Brisbane in December ready for her glorious new life. She had no idea how different that life would be — or that she was about to be diagnosed with breast cancer.

A month earlier, 3 December, she'd gone for a mammogram

through the public health system in Canberra. 'I had the test and happily moved to Brisbane two weeks later.

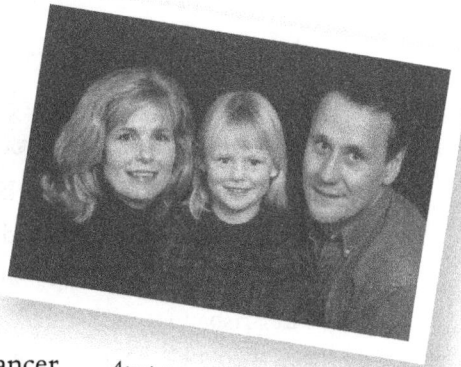
Anni, Laura and Mark

'What had happened was that on my 43rd birthday, I decided I should have a mammogram because my auntie died of breast cancer at 43. It was one of those things I thought I should do and then tick it off. Because of the ACT policy in the December period, I was asked to sign a statement that I was happy to wait to get my results in January. I think it was done with the best of intentions because that's a time when consultants are on holidays, but in my case it backfired,' she says resignedly. 'In hindsight, maybe I shouldn't have signed it, but you never believe that you have cancer, so you don't make a fuss and just gaily sign it off.'

Anni arrived in Brisbane on 19 December, and the next day she found the lump. 'We'd moved into our beautiful new home and I got stuck into the unpacking and settling in. That day we bought a Christmas tree, and Laura and I had a swim in the pool. I remember thinking how wonderful it was to be up here in the tropics. "This is the life," I had said to myself smugly.

'I went upstairs to have a shower and get changed. I bent over and thought, "Ooh, what's that?" You always wonder what a lump would feel like and this one was so big I couldn't believe that I hadn't felt it before. It was so large I thought, "That's not good," but I didn't want to spoil everyone's Christmas. My parents are in England, my sister is in Germany, and my brother lives in America — I just couldn't ruin their Christmas fun with a worrying phone call,' says Anni. 'But realising it could be serious, I also just couldn't ignore it. If it was cancerous then the sooner it was out the better. So I told my husband Mark.

'When I found the lump I immediately rang the Canberra breast cancer testing clinic to ask them for help as I didn't know what to do. I was in a new city and didn't know anyone. But that day was the Friday of their Christmas party and everyone was either out at the lunch or had left for holidays. My results would have been there and would have shown the tumour but no one was there to look at them and contact me. I was shattered and I felt it was shoddy treatment. I eventually calmed down a bit and realised I would have to deal with it here in Brisbane.

'The doctors in Canberra did contact me on 8 January to tell me I should come in straight away for more tests. But by that time I had found the lump and my treatment was well under way.'

Not knowing any local doctors, Anni and Mark looked in the *Yellow Pages*, found a General Practitioner in their suburb and went to see him. 'He turned out to be lovely, and in spite of it being the holiday period, he managed to somehow get me into the Wesley Hospital and in contact with an excellent oncologist and surgeon,' says Anni gratefully.

'We decided to leave surgery until after Christmas, so on Boxing Day I was scheduled for surgery.'

After discussions, Anni and Mark decided to tell six-year-old Laura, despite any concerns about her young age. 'We've always been very honest with her and I have a belief that you should always tell kids the truth, otherwise their imagination goes wild. Of course, it was only in basic terms but she was aware that it was serious and knew I would have to go to hospital for surgery. Gradually, over the years, she has understood more and she's handled it remarkably well — more so the older she gets.'

Anni's daughter is now 12, but it is clear that she possesses a maturity beyond her years. 'She's very stoic and has a calmness about it. She's amazing, and although she doesn't talk much about the cancer she knows she can ask me anything at any time.

'I've often tried to remember back to when I was 12 and how I dealt with any dramas — not that they were very serious — and I think kids actually take things a lot better than we imagine. We share everything with Laura — share, not burden her. We were caught out a couple of times so now we've learned to share everything and be inclusive.'

And there has been a lot to share. Anni's first diagnosis was a Grade 3 tumour which had spread to her lymph glands, necessitating the removal of 15 lymph nodes and leaving her with an ongoing problem with lymphoedema. She then went through two bouts of chemotherapy, separated by a month of radiation treatments in between.

'That evil FEC chemo cocktail was horrible. I'd have it on Thursday and I guarantee by Sunday I would be violently ill. I didn't travel well with the treatment, but being a conventional person I just accepted that it was inevitable. I thought it was obvious that I should go through it to give myself the best chance of survival.'

Reflecting on her early treatment, Anni is very grateful for not only the Herculean support which Mark provides, but the support of her oncologist, Geoffrey Beadle, whom she credits with 'getting me through everything. Emotional care is almost more important than medical,' she says. 'My medical team over the years keeps expanding, but he is always at the core of it and was always up to date. That gave me enormous confidence.'

On 9 September 2001, after nine months of treatments, Anni finally finished her medical care. 'The day I finished I was euphoric. I had come through the tunnel and all I could think of was "No more bloody pink crap!"' she laughs. 'If I could bottle that jubilation and sell it I'd be a millionaire — and it lasted for months, which was something I didn't expect.

'Having finally got through the treatments, I desperately wanted to see my family in England so I flew straight over. I landed at Heathrow on 11 September, and ours was the last plane to land on that fateful day. What a way to herald the end of chemo!' she laughs.

'I was strong, healthy, active and busy. I was back at work full time. It was all routine, but I loved feeling normal again. Everything was going really well for almost five years, until July 2005 when I started getting tweaks in my lower back. I didn't think there was anything sinister with the pain as I had strained my back earlier. I kept putting the niggles down to that strain. I had read that the cancer can return to the lower back, but I just ignored it.

'Then one day I realised that my back was bothering me and halfway through my morning walk I felt ill and wanted to vomit. Again, I passed it off as having gulped my breakfast tea and felt that it would pass. But I then thought I had better see the doctor about my back. He suggested an X-ray and of course it came back as suspect.' Anni's voice drops to a whisper. 'It was cancer to the bone and then everything snowballed with lots of tests. It was like, "Bingo, I've hit the jackpot with lots of new tumours."

'It was like a rollercoaster. I remember going into Mark's office, where the report had been sent, and he read out "suspected" and I just broke down. I was very emotional. I was not really angry; it was more absolute disappointment. But there had always been something niggling me in the back of my mind — wondering, "Is it going to come back?" After my first treatments, the doctor sent me on my merry way and we never mentioned words like remission.'

When the cancer did return, Anni went into shock and felt frustrated that after doing all the right things it had come back. 'I'd been there, done that and conquered that one — but now I had to face it again. And I do admit to beating myself up quite a bit. I knew in those past four years I'd worked too hard and taken so much on, but I'd tried very hard to keep the stress levels down because I was convinced stress was very bad for my health.'

There's a stoicism about Anni as she quietly relives those terrible days of investigations. The results showed that secondary tumours were throughout her skeleton. They had also spread into the liver and there was a large tumour in her right breast.

Needing to see her family in England, Anni again travelled home in September 2006 to make the emotionally difficult visit to her parents. It was while she was with them that she had a seizure. It was then she knew that the disease had invaded her brain. 'I did have a warning from my oncologist that because of some of the drugs I was taking that I was vulnerable to the tumours spreading to my brain. You hope it doesn't happen.'

Indeed, Anni still gets angry at herself for not mentioning her back pain earlier. 'I was still on my three-monthly visits to Dr Beadle and on my last consultation I just didn't say anything. I'd got to a stage that I felt I was always complaining about insignificant things, that I was being neurotic and imagining pains and problems. I felt I was becoming a hypochondriac so I said nothing. Now I tell everyone whenever I can, "If you have any pain, no matter how slight, you go to the doctor,"' she tells me firmly.

This drive to help others survive breast cancer is a passion, which is why 'Mark and I are both members of the National Breast Cancer Foundation's volunteer speakers' bureau.

'I know that the drugs that I'm on are what keeps me alive — and it is only through funding research that we are going to find a cure for this terrible disease,' she says.

Indeed, so committed is she to the cause that she had a pink ribbon tattooed onto her right arm. 'My older brother, Johnny, lives in America and has a few tattoos. When I was in England in 2006 he came over and wanted us to get what he called bonding tattoos. Unfortunately, I had my seizure and wasn't well enough to do that. So when he visited me here in Brisbane in April 2007 the first thing he did was to take me to get our matching tats. He has a contemporary stylised version of the pink ribbon on his wrists and he tells me that he thinks of me when he washes up,' she says, smiling and flexing her pink-ribboned bicep.

'Johnny is a high school teacher and when he went back to California he found that his students — especially the girls — appreciated the meaning of the tattoo. And it was his way of getting the awareness message out there. It was really a special thing for us to do.'

Her secondary cancer diagnosis was certainly overwhelming for Anni but she says she never loses hope. 'I think it is all about how you approach things. I am a very positive person and although both times my diagnosis was distressing, I've never panicked or thought I was going to curl up and die. I just get on with it and keep going,' she asserts.

And that included more bouts of chemotherapy. 'I was so elated the first time — knowing the terrible chemo was over — that this time I had to take sedatives before even facing chemotherapy. Because I knew how debilitating those chemo drugs were, I just couldn't go back into the bull-pit without medication.

'I don't sink into depressive moods and I am really glad I am like that.' But she acknowledges that she does have difficult moments 'like throwing up all night, and being compromised in what I can do'.

However, Anni has never considered giving up. 'I'm stubborn and I'm determined to continue going on strongly. And the further I've gone on both these journeys, I've become even more determined, more courageous and found greater strength in myself.

'My doctors have never talked timelines with me; it's never come up and I certainly don't want to know. I think if I ask, then it's like ticking off on my life, and because my life is uncertain I don't want to spend whatever time I have left just waiting to die.

'I don't want a lifetime clock for death — that's a waste of time. We can't stop it and I don't want to put any power into thinking, "Is it this week? Or this year?" So it is something I have pushed right out of my mind. I want to live in the now and use all my energy living a good life rather than just surviving.'

Anni has a Buddhist-style philosophy about her future, saying, 'Inevitably we all die and we can't stop it. That gives me a lot of calmness and peace. I am not afraid of death.'

Her positivity did take a bit of a battering when she had to spend many weeks in and out of hospital. She confesses to me that during this treatment, for the first time ever, dark thoughts intruded.

'I was so sick of being prodded and pricked, having blood taken, seeing a whole range of specialists and tests being done, that for the first time I succumbed in my weaker periods. I didn't know if I could keep this up. But then I got stronger and my resolve returned,' she adds with that determined smile. 'I look at the photo of Laura, and out at the trees and the river and know that life is still worth living.'

'I am just so proud of Laura. I visualise her milestones — the 18th and 21st birthdays, university, leaving school, boyfriends, getting married — and me being there beside her. No way am I not going to be there,' she says adamantly. 'The thought of her not having a mum is really too much to bear and breaks my heart. But it gives me the motivation to stay positive. Every day I sit and use my visualisation to see me there beside Laura at all of her significant landmarks.'

Although Anni faces major medical challenges, she speaks of them with a dismissive wave. With considerable feeling, she tells me that her greatest challenge is to be a good mum. 'Because of my frailness, Mark does everything around the house. I feel redundant; I feel useless. I wish I could be a better wife and I can hardly bear to think of how Mark would cope without me. It seems we have always been one unit and looked forward to growing old together.'

Tears well in her eyes. 'There are certain things that I just can't do, like the girly shopping at Indooroopilly, driving myself around and even cooking meals.'

But Anni does now accept that things are how they are and admits that she is guilty of 'beating myself up. It doesn't stop me wishing I could be a better mother, but I am very proud of Laura and her total support for me. I do the very best I can at the moment.'

It is the many special moments that keep Anni going; like the Mother's Day letter that Laura wrote, telling her what a wonderful mother she is. 'That almost broke my heart,' she adds. Anni also treasures the Christmas letter where Laura begged Santa to make her mother better. 'The letter said that it wasn't fair, that I was such a good person, who had already been through one bout of cancer, and that I didn't deserve another.

'Laura does, however, know her limits and if the cancer talk becomes too much she just tells me "enough". When Belinda Emmett died, I was desperate to protect Laura so at first I hid all the papers and wouldn't turn on the television. But then I realised that was silly and wasn't doing her any good,' she says.

'She knows it is a potentially fatal disease and after watching one of the news stories Laura turned to me and bluntly asked me if I was going to die. That really shook me, coming so much from left field that I didn't really know how to answer her. I obviously had to tell her I was okay; but I also had to tell her that it is a deadly disease and I just didn't know. I told her the drugs were important and are doing their job and keeping me going. But I honestly couldn't answer her; I couldn't tell her anything else. It was an extremely difficult moment.' There is a lull in our conversation, but it is short-lived.

Whilst Anni retains her optimism and is resolute in saying she's not done yet, she does own up to concerns about how her health is holding up. 'It is disappointing that I am on my fourth lot of chemotherapy now and the drugs seem to be losing their efficacy. I've had several unpleasant side effects, like numbness, losing my toenails and the skin on my feet. That's a bit worrying, but my doctors tell me there are still lots of options.'

One of the life lessons that Anni feels she has learned well is the value of time. 'Time is really precious. And I now realise how important it is. I was pretty much a workaholic. I don't think I neglected Laura but as long as she was okay I kept working. She's never been a clinging child and has always been independent, but with hindsight I realise that I was working too hard.

'After my initial diagnosis I felt an urgency to do so much, reaching all those goals and trying to tick off as many of life's experiences as possible. I was doing a floristry course, doing a university degree and working at a full-on job. I was so determined to get to the top, I was really working too hard and too long. But with the second diagnosis I stopped. I realised that time is too precious to do all of those things, and the reality is that I physically can't do them now.'

Anni wants to use her experience to make a difference for others. One of her main ambitions in this regard is to see the implementation of a body awareness element in schools' sex education program that includes teaching girls to check their breasts. 'My next move is to lobby Education Queensland to get that idea incorporated into the program. I see it as a clever way to save lives. We all think we are too young or that we won't be the ones who get breast cancer so an increased awareness, starting when girls are young, is something I dearly want to get moving.'

Our chat is drawing to an end. Ever-positive, Anni tells me she has no time for dark reflections. 'What's done is done. I move forward, live for today and enjoy each and every day — smelling the roses, as they say.'

I drive away uplifted and inspired by Anni Franklin Wood, whose gentle wisdom and optimistic philosophy encourages me to see my own life through her wonderfully rose-tinted glasses. I vow to live my future one special day at a time.

POSTSCRIPT
EMAIL: 9 DECEMBER 2007

Anni had a wonderful time over her extended 50th birthday weekend. Since then Anni's health has deteriorated considerably; she spent a week in hospital, where she finally lost consciousness. On Monday we made the decision to bring her home, as she had requested. She is surrounded by all her favourite things in the world, including flowers, photographs, beloved pets and most importantly constant love and caring. She is unable to speak, but is clearly aware of being home. We are still hoping and praying for a miracle, but are realistic about the situation.

As always, our darling Laura is an inspiration. She is coping so well with this situation, which for any age is hard, but as a 12-year-old may be even harder. I am so proud, as I know Anni is.

Mark Wood

EMAIL: 14 DECEMBER 2007

Anni is at peace, with no more pain. She passed away at home in my arms at 6.20pm on 12 December 2007. We are so proud of her. She was and will always be the love of our lives.

Mark and Laura Wood

Hello everyone!

Today I started my radiotherapy: one down, 32 to go. For the next seven weeks (three off days) I have radiotherapy each week day. The end seems like eons away, but so did chemo and I survived that.

By the second week in December this will be just a memory! I'll then have two weeks until I finish work and get ready for the best Christmas of my life. Cancer-free, two of the most beautiful tiny girls in the world, family and friends. Don't need Christmas presents with those gifts.

Radiotherapy seems pretty easy — lie on a bed, get zapped, get up from the bed. I understand it is very draining and by the end I will be very tired, but it helps that I can plan for that. I go at 3.30ish each day and then go home, so I can have a catnap and catch up on energy and still occasionally have that Christmas party night out!!!

In fact, after radiotherapy today I booked in for a Chinese massage — bliss. I felt that I needed to combine these two from the start so that I make sure I get the rest I need — and any excuse to lie down and relax!

The other good thing about radiotherapy is that it doesn't make me sick. The joys of food are returning quickly. After 162 days of feeling sick to a greater or lesser degree, it is such a pleasure to eat my favourite foods again. In fact, to mark this new stage, I arrived home to find the bubbly was cold and a dozen plump oysters waiting. Pete had also cooked a roast dinner for us.

Now — if only I could lose the weight I've put on with chemo and get all the tufts of hair to gel together I'd be happy. Actually, I really am happy. I'm on the final stretch, and with your continued support (not long now) the time will fly and we'll all be toasting 2004 with Moet.

Keep smiling

AM

Carole Haddad's Journey

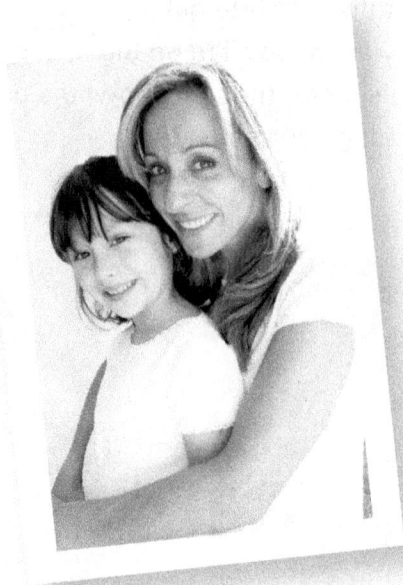

'I tell [people] I've done the Kokoda. They think I've been to New Guinea, but I've never been there. Every form I filled in during my radiation treatment, I'd cross out the C for Cancer and put K for Kokoda because everything I did was like going through my own personal Kokoda challenge.'

I meet Carole Haddad at her trendy hair salon at Brisbane's Southbank. After giving a client's hair a final buff, she sweeps through the salon, her high-octane energy buzzing, to attend to business before our interview. The now beautifully coiffured client whispers to me, 'Isn't she amazing? We were all there for her because we love Carole and admired the way she kept on going. So please be gentle with her.'

Carole is still very raw. She finished treatment only weeks ago and the emotional floodgates open often during our chat. But beneath the fragility of this vibrant lady is a strong determination to live a long and valuable life, unhindered by anything like a diagnosis of cancer.

Carole's experience was also made harder because she is a fiercely independent single mother to daughter Priscilla and, although supported in her journey by friends, she acknowledges, 'I was responsible for my own life. I was really the only one who could help me.'

'The C word — isn't that Carole?' she says as we begin to talk.

Before her diagnosis, Carole wasn't in a good space. In her own words, her life was 'hectic, frenetic. I was worried all the time, mostly about silly things. I was trying to do everything for everyone, make everyone else happy. There was no balance in my life and I was feeling negative about myself.'

In late 2006, Carole had a sense that something just wasn't right in her life — many women found to have breast cancer talk about having a similar feeling before diagnosis. For several months before she found the lump, she seemed often to notice books and articles about breast cancer, and felt compelled to read them. 'I'd read about Kylie and Belinda and I'd ask myself what am I doing reading this stuff for?

'Then one night I was lying in bed watching one of those hospital reality TV shows and it sort of prompted me to check my breasts. And that's when I found the lump. I freaked out. For the next two hours until midnight I stood in front of the mirror and looked at that lump. It was obvious,' she says.

Carole woke next morning to see if her nightmare was actually true. 'I got up thinking this isn't real; this is going to go away. But I could still see the lump and my heart fell to the floor.'

Carole was in denial: it took her two days to book in to see her GP. Her doctor explained that because Carole had breast implants, it wasn't a sinister lump, just hormonal, and that everything was fine. But Carole knew in her heart that all wasn't right so she asked for a referral to a surgeon.

'I know in my heart when I've had hard decisions to make or when I compete in international hairdressing competitions, there's a nerve, that funny feeling that tells me something is wrong. Sitting there that day I knew things weren't going to go well for me,' she says.

When the surgeon told her that indeed the lump didn't look good, she was distressed but grateful that she'd listened to her gut instinct and sought a second opinion. But the earliest appointment for a mammogram and biopsy was not for another three weeks — 19 December. 'I just bawled. I just knew I wasn't going to have a good Christmas. Even though the surgeon said to think positively, I just knew it was bad news.'

She somehow got through those three weeks and went for the ultrasound. It showed shadows; this meant I had to have a biopsy. 'I was crying uncontrollably. The nurses were lovely, telling me that it would be okay. But it wasn't. I felt I had just died, that my body had gone to a war zone.

'I was supposed to ring my doctor for the results, but I just couldn't. I was numb. Eventually, next day he rang me and told me to come in urgently. I dragged myself across the road to his surgery and he told me the biopsy showed breast cancer.

'I just collapsed. I literally fell in a heap on the floor. I couldn't speak. The doctor told me it was a DCIS [ductal carcinoma in situ] but I couldn't understand anything he was saying. All I could think of was that I was going to die.'

As it is just Carole and her daughter Priscilla at home, Carole asked her close friend, Alfie, to come with her to the specialist because 'I knew I wouldn't hear anything properly. I knew I needed an interpreter with me so she could take notes, understand what I had to do.

'I rang Alfie about ten times a day for the next week asking her questions about what I was supposed to do. You can't ring your doctor every hour or so, so it was so wonderful to be able to talk with her.'

Because she felt she needed to be as informed as possible, Carole read every book she could get her hands on, but nothing sunk in. She was in a whirlwind of fear and lack of knowledge.

Carole hadn't told six-year-old Priscilla what was happening, but somehow her daughter just knew something was wrong. The night before Carole was scheduled for her operation, she had an epiphany.

'Priscilla and I were lying in bed. We always pray before she goes to sleep, so I prayed and then I said, 'It's your turn.' Priscilla simply said, "Please, Jesus, make my mummy better."

'I couldn't sleep all night. I cried my heart out and several hours later I realised no one could help me out of this. I was looking all around me for the answers then suddenly I understood that the answer was right with me. Basically, it's me. I am the only answer. I finally comprehended that the outcome is in my hands. I alone could change anything,' she says.

'I also realised that prior to my diagnosis I had probably lost a bit of faith in myself and my ability to do things right. Now I had my confidence in me back. And finally I slept.'

Carole sprang out of bed next morning and vowed that she wasn't going to die, that this wasn't the end for her. 'I was going to attack the cancer like a tiger. All my life I have battled and now I have too many good things in my life to give up.

'When I woke from the op. the doctor held my hand and spoke the magic words: "I got it all and it is not invasive. It is only DCIS." I was so lucky — the breast implants had pushed the lump up so I had found it early before it went into the ducts.

'I went home that afternoon. I was so grateful, so alive that I couldn't sleep for two days. I kept thinking and thinking about how I had to change my life — everything had to change for the better. It was empowering. I am so grateful I found my life!

'I knew my daughter was precious to me and I realised how much I love my work. No one was going to destroy what was great in my life. I came to realise that I needed to de-stress, take the load off my shoulders and make things right in my life for the future.

'I came into my salon the day after the op. — which shocked everyone. But they were even more surprised when I sacked eight people that morning. I just could not have gone through radiation treatment with those eight people in my salon. They were carrying too much baggage. It was nothing to do with their work; it had to do with their personal stuff they were bringing into work. I was so in tune with myself that I was feeling all that negativity and I just had to get it out. So I cleaned the shop out. Over the next month I got a new team.'

Carole's determination to take absolute control of her life saw her in the shop every day; she didn't have a single day off. Each day she would cut, colour and style. 'I was so organised that I could put on a colour for a client, dash off around the corner to the Mater Hospital for a quick "zap" and be back in time to rinse the colour out and blow dry the client's hair. How's that for organisation?' she laughs.

Actually, many of her regulars had twigged to the fact that something was a little different. Carole has a giggle as she recounts the story of one client, who asked where she went while the colour was setting. 'When I told her I'd gone to get my radiation treatment, she said, "You have to be kidding me — no one does that!"'

But Carole did this every day for two months — remaining positive, energetic and full of hope.

However, as is the case with most women diagnosed with a serious illness, not everything was rosy for her. 'Although I was feeling good about myself, I did lose lots of friends and acquaintances along the way. Too many people think that cancer hops, skips and jumps from us to them. I was totally shocked and disappointed. But I came to realise that they were just what I now call "fashion friends" — in this year, out the next. It hurts when people you think you know can't even ask if you are okay.'

One of the most confronting examples of this was the 'date' Carole was due to meet on the day she discovered her lump. 'He obviously found out I potentially had cancer and to this day I have never heard from him. It was not as if I was going to be able to go out, but I would have thought a simple call to enquire about my health wasn't too much to ask. What am I — damaged goods?' she says, waving her hand to emphasise her point.

'When I have had clients or friends diagnosed, I have always been supportive — shaving heads, getting wigs or just letting them talk, which destroys me emotionally. But we owe it to people to be there for them. So to have him and other people close to me just turn their backs on me is unbelievable. What are we here on Earth for?'

Carole really can't understand how people could just wipe her out of their life when she was down and needed help. She felt she had to stay strong and positive for Priscilla. 'I couldn't burden a six-year-old, for goodness sake. But you sometimes do need to talk and release the pain and emotion — that is where friends sticking by me would have been terrific.'

She says that in fact it was strangers who supported her. 'The people who stepped up were mostly acquaintances, and now I value them as friends. That's surely what life is about.'

As well as having her hairdressing salon, Carole is part-owner in another beauty business, and she concedes that her dealings with her partner during her treatment caused her more angst than she could cope with at the time.

'We had to meet to discuss business lots of times, and I was so easily upset it became extremely difficult for him. He is only a young man. He didn't want my baggage and he couldn't cope with my hypersensitive state. The emotion was too much.

'But the interesting thing was that as much as he didn't want to deal with that side of my illness, he really would do anything for me. And, funnily enough, he was the one scouring the papers and magazines for any relevant articles on breast cancer. So in fact he did care, he just didn't know how to show it. That was another lesson I learned — that men struggle a lot and don't cope well with the emotional toll that cancer brings with it,' Carole adds.

She now sees the world with new eyes. 'My life is completely different,' is how she puts it. She has a new team at work, she is no longer stressed, she worries less and claims her energy levels have skyrocketed since she 'attacked this disease like a tiger'. She sleeps well these days, is hungry for work and feels a happiness and contentment in her life that takes her breath away.

'I realise that I have a huge life that I wasn't living for me. So now I take time out to spend quality time with my precious daughter, Priscilla. I am enjoying every single day. I laugh so much now that stress has no part in this new life. I am definitely happier,' she says, adding cheekily, 'except for the man situation!'

Carole then becomes contemplative and silently reflects on the past six months before saying, 'When people ask me what I've been doing, I tell them I've done the Kokoda. They think I've been to New Guinea, but I've never been there. Every form I filled in during my radiation treatment, I'd cross out the C for Cancer and put K for Kokoda because everything I did was like going through my own personal Kokoda challenge.'

Carole approached her radiation with such positive zeal that even if she'd needed to have chemotherapy, she says she'd have done it. 'Heck, I would have done anything to make sure it was gone and I would stay alive. I'd still beat it.'

Looking towards her future, Carole enthusiastically lists some of the many things she still wants to do before she dies. 'I want to see my daughter grow up; I want to do her hair for her wedding. And I haven't yet cut Madonna's hair!

'I've still got so much left to achieve,' she says softly. The rawness of her experience then unleashes more tears, prompting her to ask me not to think her silly and too sensitive. On the contrary, I am drawn to comfort her, recognising the deep emotional impact that breast cancer causes.

For the past six years Carole has worked with Gretel Killeen on the reality TV show *Big Brother*. She developed a close professional relationship with Gretel but was totally unprepared for the support that she received from the *BB* star.

'I couldn't believe it. Gretel was overseas and she rang me the day of my operation. Here's a woman I just worked with — it's just my job, although we did form a friendship — and she's on the other side of the world. She picked up the phone and rang me. She told me I should just grab the challenge by the balls and fight. Even at rehearsal on the opening night of *Big Brother*, when she saw me, she stopped and came over to ask if I was okay. That was just so wonderful. She did for me what many of my so-called friends couldn't do — simply ask how I was.'

As Carole sits, thinking about the many kindnesses that people offered, her assistant gently interrupts to tell her that the shop is full and could she please come as everyone is waiting for her magic fingers. After a quick wipe of the eyes and a flick of the hair, with shoulders straightened, Carole is back to her salon and her work.

She is putting away the emotional challenge of her breast cancer until tonight when, lying down next to Priscilla as her daughter goes to sleep, she says a prayer of gratitude — as she does each night — that she is still alive to step up for all those as yet unfulfilled dreams.

Hello Lovely FOAMs

Can you believe it is November and therefore close to
Christmas? Time when you look ahead seems like it will take
forever — especially if something wonderful lies at the end.
This year has moved much faster than I thought. In May, I
knew it would travel slowly and I'd be glad when it had gone.
Then I realised that I would then be wishing away an important
part of my life and my history and who I am, so I have been
grateful that I have kept a diary chronicling this part of my life.

Otherwise I may have forgotten little joys like the Breast
Cancer Fashion Parade. It was a special night. Not because
I got to wear clothes that each cost as much as a trip to
England, but because it allowed me to be absorbed into a sea
of support and love at a time I really needed friends and love.

Chemo has added about 7kgs to my small frame, the
radiotherapy is leaving burn marks, my skin is mottled, and
my hair is just starting to appear and it's dark! But none of
that matters when people, most of whom you have never
met, can lighten your soul with a smile, a hug or a word
of encouragement. Many of the audience were survivors
of cancer, but many were there to just give us a symbolic
emotional hug to keep on going.

If I rushed through this period I may not have appreciated
how cancer can wonderfully give you a glimpse into the joy
of living, like when Anthony spoke yesterday. Anthony's little

5-year-old daughter Sarah has cancer and is 'the face' of the Children's Hospital Foundation's Christmas Appeal.

I had organised a corporate Christmas thank you for the RCHF sponsors and asked Anthony to say thank you on behalf of all the sick kids like Sarah. He spoke of his 'walk through the valley of darkness' and the terror of holding his daughter's limp body after chemo. I sobbed through his address (as did even some of the most hardened businessmen) but I couldn't help feeling the importance of living a joyous life and being grateful for God allowing me to come through.

But my magic moment came at the end of the breakfast, when Sarah and I sat chatting and laughing and she leaned over to me and took off her signature purple hat, stroked my head and offered to share her hat. Her mum told me it had never come off and absolutely no one is allowed wear it.

We've all read *The Purple Hat* story that is often circulated via email. It has always symbolised for me the freedom of growing old disgracefully and being our best selves. How could Sarah's gift not be a special milestone for me when a 5-year-old can show such empathy! A moment I will carry with me to my grave. Thank you, Sarah. Such joy for living in that little girl is contagious and I am humbled and blessed to be 'Sarah's friend'.

I've still got another five weeks of radiotherapy. But Vanesa comes up this week for her birthday so I can look forward to sharing special family days with her, Ben, Kylie and the gorgeous Mads and Ella.

Now, if I can only go and find my own purple hat, I'll be right ...

Smiling still

AM

Kitty Lyons' Journey

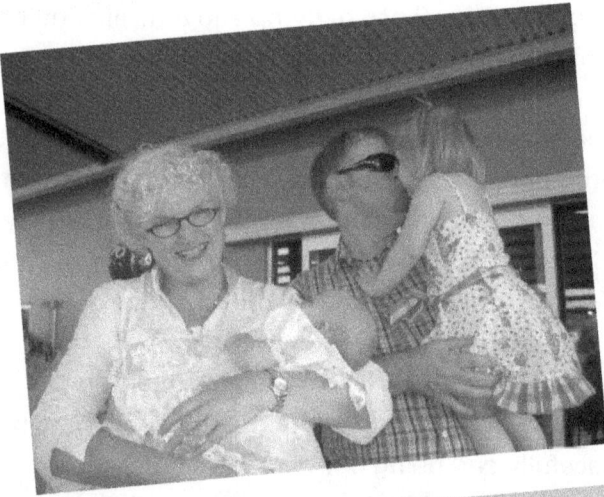

'Before cancer, my attitude was, "Life is a bitch and then you die," but having cancer forced me into realising that I really know nothing about death but that I have life — and that without me honouring my own existence and my own life, there is no point in living.'

itty Lyons sees her battle with breast cancer more as a voyage of discovery within herself and her soul than as a physical journey. Whilst she was fighting the breast cancer disease with traditional medical treatments, the true triumph for Kitty was the emotional and spiritual victory in changing her attitude to life. During our meeting, she declares more than once that breast cancer was the best thing to happen to her.

Kitty explains that in 2001, when she was diagnosed, hers was a difficult life and she had no expectation that things could be any other way for her. 'I believed my life was tough and, in fact, I have always thought life was meant to be tough. It was an attitude I grew up with and it had become my truth.

'In my late twenties I married and, some years later, had two wonderful children. Unfortunately, my husband had a few issues relating to money management, which caused us to bump along the bottom financially for many years. Most of the time we lurched from one crisis to another. I found myself using all of my energy in crisis management and not taking the time to reflect or deal with the real issues.

'Whenever there was an emotional problem, I avoided it. I used to tell myself that I couldn't work it out at the time so I'd think about it later. That left me feeling constantly uncertain. My husband had a very good heart. He was my friend and was charming and warm, and on a day-to-day basis it was wonderful. But then there was the gambling, which created huge problems. It is not just money that these addictive people gamble with. They are risk-takers and they gamble with your love, your life, your emotions and even your relationships,' Kitty explains.

Then in 1998, Kitty's husband died of melanoma after a four-year battle with the disease, leaving Kitty a single mum of 46 with six- and eight-year-old sons.

'On my husband's death I was, on the one hand, filled with so much grief at the loss of my soul mate, but at the same time I was almost angry with myself at being sad at losing this man who had caused me so much pain. I was left in debt to bring up two young sons. But I managed — just.'

Kitty moved from the Gold Coast to Boonah, a pretty country town an hour's drive from Brisbane, nestled in the Scenic Rim just beyond Ipswich. She bought a house and felt a deep personal pride growing in her as she moved from the very co-dependent relationship with her late husband to a new, independent life.

'Being able to stand on my own two feet and establish myself as a single person, making important decisions like moving and buying a house whilst also looking after young children, was an enormous, absolutely enormous, challenge for me,' says Kitty.

Even though she took pride in her achievements, life again became tough for Kitty. Then, when she was diagnosed with breast cancer three years later, life was about as challenging as it gets. 'There is an energy within, which, over the years, I had drawn upon to help me deal with each crisis as it unfolded, but eventually it ran out,' she says sadly.

'I don't really understand it, but I think this was my life energy and I just used it all up. I am very careful not to go near that place now. If anything gets too difficult or too hard, I am not ever going to touch that well of energy.

'When I reflect on why I got breast cancer, I believe it was an accumulation of many things: it was the way I dealt with grief over my husband's death; it was continually delving into my energy well; and it was a feeling that life was just too tough for me. I remember one day driving on the highway, and from very deep within me came a feeling of release. I felt, "I will be glad to go."'

This really frightened Kitty because she didn't understand where this sense of despair, of welcoming death, came from. 'It wasn't that I didn't want to live but I just felt life was too difficult for me to cope with.' She believes that to pull her up from that dark place, it required something of the seriousness of a life-threatening disease like breast cancer. 'This was the only thing that could save me. And it did,' she says.

Approximately 18 months after her husband died, Kitty found a lump in her breast. Because she was dealing with her grief, she didn't do anything about it for another 18 months. 'When I realised the lump was still there, I wasn't really worried but felt that I'd prefer it out rather than in,' says Kitty.

Rather than being daunting, the prospect of going to hospital for surgery was almost enticing as it entailed a form of respite for her. 'The image of lying on a bed for 24 hours — of being looked after and not having to look after the kids and deal with my everyday problems — was wonderful.

'I thought the removal of the lump would be purely housekeeping — until I got the dreadful call from the doctor saying the pre-surgery tests had detected some suspect cells. I was in a car park at the shopping centre. I had my arms full of groceries and the kids were walking with me. I knew then my life was changed from that very moment,' she says emphatically.

Immediately Kitty was off to hospital, where the surgeon operated and removed the cancerous tissue. The biopsy showed that the lump was malignant and that the surgical margins for the tumour had not been wide enough.

'When I was diagnosed, I went on a search for alternative therapies. I went to a number of different practitioners: naturopaths, kinesiologists, spiritual people. I had decided that I wasn't going to have chemotherapy or radiotherapy. I've always done things with alternative medicine and I was convinced that was the pathway for me to follow,' says Kitty.

'On this whole tour of natural therapies, I was looking for someone to tell me that this was going to have a good outcome; that I was going to be okay. Finally, I found a naturopath whom I felt was on the right track. He approached healing in a scientific way which included both conventional medicine and alternative treatments and did seem to have proven results. But his treatments were going to cost me $400 each month. When my husband got sick, we did not have the financial resources to pay for alternative treatment, and I had promised myself that I would never allow this to happen to my family again.

'But this was my life on the line and I didn't have the funds to buy the medicine so I really had no choice but to rely on conventional methods.'

Unfortunately, the surgeon had gone on holiday, leaving Kitty wondering what she should do next. Knowing that the lump had been malignant, she went to see another surgeon to organise more surgery to clear the margins and to remove the glands. 'But I didn't want to have my glands taken out, so the surgeon cut out a much wider margin and, in doing so, discovered another whole group of cancerous cells. He rang me to say that it wasn't looking good and that he should take the breast off. And then he, too, went on holiday,' Kitty says in amazement. 'Both took holidays after giving me bad news, which was difficult in itself to deal with.

'So I went back to the first surgeon, who had now returned from his break. He assured me that the initial lump had been taken out completely and that I was very lucky that I had gone to the other doctor. This first surgeon told me that on his reading of the results, he would not have put me back into surgery.

'By this time I was totally shattered and I didn't have a clue about what I should do. Here I was, coming to a doctor to have my breast off, and he says that he doesn't think I need to. I didn't know what was right or wrong, which way was up or down. I was completely lost,' Kitty says.

During this emotional time, Kitty had to try to remain calm so that she could work out what she needed to do. She knew she had to make important decisions about her future.

'After thinking about all of the confusing information, I basically came to the conclusion that I needed to fight this on all fronts. I needed to fight it through conventional medicine: burn it out, poison it, cut it out — whatever it takes to live,' she said decisively. 'I knew that it was fear-motivated, but that was where I was at that time.'

The surgeon convinced Kitty that she did not need a mastectomy.

So Kitty did keep her breast but had to go through an extensive program of chemotherapy and radiotherapy. Each treatment entailed an arduous 200km round trip from Boonah to Brisbane.

'Of course, this was daunting. Here I was, a single mother of two boys aged nine and 11. Recently, one of the boys told me that he didn't understand what was going on then. Which was fine with me — I didn't want them to worry or be unnecessarily affected by what was happening to me, but at the same time I spoke openly with them and did not try to be secretive.

'Bless my mother. She made a huge effort. She came and stayed with us for about three days each time I had chemo. She helped me out financially, paying for my treatments. But I still have no idea how I coped.'

Kitty shakes her head in disbelief as she recalls the kindnesses of her country community. She continues to be amazed by the generosity of the people of Boonah. 'The local community is largely Christian, and they offered an immense amount of help. I didn't know many of them, but they spread the word around that I needed help and so they rallied around helping me in so many ways. One woman came every Friday and vacuumed my house; others cooked. All the churches had me on their prayer lists,' she says with gratitude.

'The school teacher of one of my boys dropped around every month I was on chemo with a pot of wheatgrass. Wheatgrass is very expensive, but he didn't ask for a cent, and half the time I didn't even see him drop it off. My neighbours came over just before Christmas and gave me $70 in cash to buy presents for the boys.

'The RSL had a wonderful community service that subsidised taxi fares to Brisbane for medical treatments. That really helped me a lot and enabled me to get to the city for my treatments. The Cancer Council also helped. They paid my major bills, which enabled me to get by.

'It made such a difference to me because there had been some talk about putting my children in care, which was just absolutely shattering. I couldn't imagine that my kids would be in care.

'The assistance I received was quite extraordinary,' Kitty says. 'I received many, many acts of kindness from all sorts of people that I was unaware I had any impact on their lives.'

Although undertaking the standard medical treatments, Kitty continued her quest for alternative healing. She read every book she could find and came to the ultimate conclusion that in every facet of healing there must be recognition of the creative force and your own physiological processes. She found kinesiology to be very helpful. She linked up with a mentor and, with his help and education, Kitty started to completely re-evaluate her life.

'My whole outlook on life changed. I could now believe that the universe loved me and that I am not here alone to have to fight my battles. I discovered that the universe applauds when human beings become conscious of their divinity.

'There is a whole joy knowing that the universe is applauding you — and believing it! I have studied the teachings of Prem Rawat, known as Maharaji, for the past 30 years but I never quite believed it until now. He teaches a way of turning your senses inside and focusing on the essence of life — the energy of life. It is a tangible, rock-solid foundation of joy — which I had managed to compromise by feeling that life is really tough.

'My whole view of life flipped to one of living in joy and an understanding that the challenges of life don't have to rob me of the experience of my soul being nourished. Then began the healing which takes place on all levels. Diet was very important — I became highly motivated. I took it to the absolute limit. No sugar or dairy passed my lips.'

When she was diagnosed, Kitty felt she was in a place of total despair and bewilderment. Three nights after being told she had cancer, Kitty says she woke up and realised that she was still breathing and wasn't dead yet. 'I told myself to get this into perspective. I knew that if I had any chance of recovering, I had to choose life. So I knew that whatever life threw at me I would embrace it — good or bad.'

The decision to live meant that Kitty had to undertake some

really deep soul-searching. 'I really put everything out on the table about what choices I had and what I was going to do. Some religious faiths offer spiritual healing, which was absolutely attractive to me. This was definitely what I wanted; I wanted this thing to go away and be fixed.

'I thought to myself, "If I've got five years to live, or five months to live or even five minutes to live — what do I want to do with that time?" I realised I had two main options. First, I could spend this precious time begging for healing, which may or may not happen. Or I could concentrate and put my attention into appreciating and being grateful for every breath I take, and therefore experience the gift of life, through the techniques taught to me by Prem Rawat,' Kitty explains.

'And it was overwhelmingly obvious to me that being gifted with life was the place to be.

'Although that was what I really wanted, there was an equally powerful desire for someone to take away the responsibility from me. I know I chose the tougher alternative — the real option — and that was empowering. It gave me control of my own life.

'I was certainly considering the children in this decision to live — leaving them without any parent was more tragic than I could contemplate. Even so, if I was going to choose to live based on mothering my children, that choice didn't acknowledge my life as a woman, as a human being. It didn't honour my own life, and that's what needed to be respected,' she says thoughtfully.

Having decided to grab life with both hands, Kitty then struggled as she tried to reconcile the alternative therapies and philosophies with conventional medicine and treatments. Kitty realised that it all boiled down to her need to fight the cancer on all fronts with everything that was available to her. Her philosophy was to protect and to support her body as much as possible whilst going through the aggressive chemical treatments. Now, looking back, Kitty can't really say what actually cured her. She acknowledges that every level of emotional, spiritual, medical and physical support was important.

'Radiation wasn't as difficult as chemotherapy because I could fit it into the school days. I would leave Boonah when the kids went to school and be back home when they got out of school, although a couple of times I had to ring my neighbour to collect them and feed them.

'Without dramatising it, throughout the treatments I knew that I had to get dinner cooked and ready by five o'clock each night because by five I was ready to collapse in a heap.'

Once all the formal treatments of surgery, chemotherapy and radiation therapy were over, Kitty was put onto the drug Tamoxifen for the next five years. 'For three years on the drug I had the most appalling hot flushes and all the other annoying menopausal side effects. I was sick of it and in the end I couldn't take it any more. My doctor just said to give it up — which I gladly did,' she says.

The end of medical treatments and the cessation of regular medical support often ushers in a time of anxiety and worry for women. Kitty, however, found an acceptance without fear.

'At first I was a little frightened that the cancer may return, but now I have absolutely no fear. I have no doubt that my cancer was emotionally based and I am very confident that I have dealt with those issues and made the changes that needed to be made.

'On the other front, if the breast cancer came back again, I think I would deal with it very differently. I'd be much more resolved and pragmatic about accepting my lot. I am stronger and deal with life in a much more positive way.

'It seems funny, but I think getting breast cancer was the best thing that ever happened to me,' Kitty says with a chuckle. 'It focused me. It was a deep journey of facing my own mortality, and then a realisation of what life really meant to me and what was important to me. And, conversely, that showed me what was unimportant in my life.'

This was a major change in Kitty's perspective on life. 'Before cancer, my attitude was, "Life is a bitch and then you die," but having cancer forced me into realising that I really know nothing about death but that I have life — and that without me honouring my own existence and my own life, there is no point in living,' she says matter-of-factly. 'And that is certainly worth celebrating!'

Kitty has now found a new lease of life with a very different outlook. She has a much more relaxed attitude these days and is in a new relationship that is fun and makes her smile. In her own words, her once very particular diet regime is now 'more relaxed'.

She believes she has the techniques, through the teachings of Prem Rawat, to realise an optimistic and bright future. And although she says she always had those skills, it is only now, after her journey with cancer, that she has shifted her focus and found the key to truly open up her life.

'I'm in a space now where I know there is nothing fair and just about life. I have no control over my life and that's okay. I have two teenage kids; I am working to make enough to look after those kids and the house and I'm back at nursing,' Kitty says simply. 'This stage of my life is a special one. In that sense I am grateful that I am now strong enough to be my own person and to make my own decisions in my own time.

'Now I am happy. I acknowledge and honour my own existence; I am important, valuable, and worthy of being nourished. A heart filled with joy and appreciation is the highest achievement in life. It is said that you come in to life empty-handed, but I do not believe that you have to leave empty-handed. Life truly is a gift no matter how long we have it. I am living mine with a full heart!'

I just wanted to share something. My lovely uncle died yesterday of cancer. We had shared lots of experiences — none of them ones we would have chosen to have, but nevertheless did. He was very down about his cancer, feeling he would never get through it, and so I spent lots of time telling him we would fight together and raise a glass of champagne at Christmas in the faces of our disease. Sadly, I know now, he didn't believe enough and he graciously accepted his time on earth was spent. However, the joy is that he had a priest and my dad there with him as he 'just went to sleep'.

It is a big wake-up call for me. Although I know that there are huge differences, it is one of those life jolts that tells us to enjoy every day as a special one and to tell all those that you love how special they are.

So, with purple hat on my head, I say thank you to you all for your love and friendship. May we continue raising our glasses for many, many more Christmases!

Smile

AM

Jodie O'Keeffe Shares Beverley Whitfield's Journey

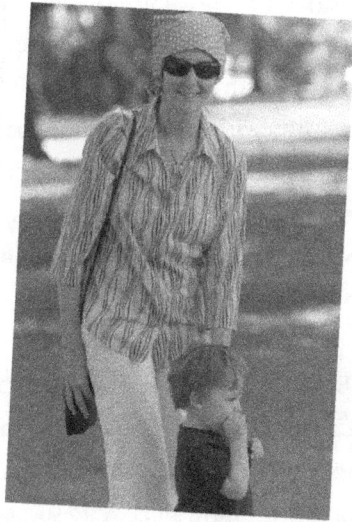

'In 2005, with Kylie Minogue's diagnosis, breast cancer was everywhere — on TV, in newspapers and magazines. I was a little cynical at that time, because everyone was so upbeat and positive about Kylie recovering, but a lot of women die.'

'I try not to be morbid, but I am not expecting a long life,' says Jodie O'Keeffe when we sit to share her mother, Beverley Whitfield's, story.

'Mum was only 57 when she died. She was a secondary school teacher, for ever and ever, and a great mum to her four kids.'

I had worked very closely with Jodie at the 2006 Melbourne Commonwealth Games and we quickly developed a personal friendship that made working together fun. However, on several occasions during that month of frenetic athletic events, I sensed a sadness, a vulnerability and a melancholy in Jodie that sometimes came upon her, but was always quickly dismissed.

It was only many months later, in one of our catch-up email chats, that she mentioned her mother had died the year before from breast cancer. She said she hadn't told me earlier so I wouldn't lose hope. This empathy and kindness was born from a year of helping her mother die peacefully, with love, dignity and no regrets.

Jodie shares her story because she believes that in our society, we don't deal with death well, even though it is a fact of life. 'If we can talk about it, and if possible prepare for death, then those who remain will be better able to cope,' she says.

When Beverley was first diagnosed in 1999, it didn't come as a complete surprise. Beverley's mother had died of breast cancer at 52 and, although Jodie feels that it probably did haunt her, she says, 'Mum never let on, although she had to have mammograms earlier than most people. A statistic I have since read suggests that one in four daughters will develop the disease and Mum, as one of four girls, was the unlucky one.'

Jodie realises she has a statistically high chance of getting breast cancer, but remains philosophical. 'I've got two sisters, and I feel a real risk as it seems to run in the maternal line. It's a comforting thought that, when I get to the vulnerable age, technology may have uncovered a cure. In my work as a journalist I report on advances in detection and treatment — so there is always hope. But, whatever happens, happens. I just don't live my life thinking I am going to be an 80-year-old,' she admits.

Jodie tries to give her daughter, Ruby, a sense of hope, even though she still feels the loss of her grandmother keenly.

'Ruby was just four years old when Kylie Minogue was diagnosed, three months after Mum died, and she was convinced Kylie would also die. So, last year I took her to Kylie's concert to show her that breast cancer isn't always a terminal illness. That gave her another, more positive, perspective.'

Beverley had found the lump herself. Tucked under her arm, it wasn't detected by mammogram, but an ultrasound and biopsy confirmed the tumour was cancerous. Jodie says her mum was a woman of her generation and she didn't talk about it much. She didn't want to worry any of her children with her feelings; her focus was on the treatment.

At that time Jodie was living overseas in London, so she doesn't really know how her mother felt emotionally. 'She wouldn't burden us with her feelings; she just carried on matter-of-factly. I had already planned to come home for holidays around that time, so fortunately I was there for the lumpectomy surgery. This was a good thing for both of us. It reassured me that she would be okay.'

However, Jodie had to return to London while her mother went through a gruelling bout of chemotherapy followed by radiation. 'It was a terrible time. I felt helpless and often, when I tried to talk with her on the phone, I could just tell she didn't have the energy. I learned to time my calls with her good days in between chemo sessions when she felt strong enough to talk. It was emotional for me being so far away, but I was confident she would come through it all.'

The family was very stoic — no doom and gloom — and their spirits were up. Beverley would finish treatment and everything would go back to normal.

In the following few years Beverley fully recovered from her treatment and was enjoying the delights of four new grandchildren.

Jodie had returned to live in Melbourne and she remembers her mother revelling in her new-found life.

'We had a couple of wonderful years. Mum really appreciated living; she was always visiting us, spending as much time as possible playing with her grandkids.

'Mum really thought she had the cancer beaten, but she still made the most of every second she had. She didn't verbalise it, and there was no impending gloom, but perhaps she had a sense that her life could be short,' says Jodie.

Beverley had tremendous faith in the medical profession. 'She took her Tamoxifen religiously. Once she was at my house in Melbourne and had forgotten to bring her tablet. Instead of staying the night, she drove the 95-minute trip back to her home in the country town of Murchison to take it. She followed the doctor's orders as a way of protecting herself from any secondary cancer.'

But it wasn't to be.

In November 2003, Jodie's father, Desmond, was dispatched to each of the family to tell them that Beverley had been diagnosed with a secondary cancer in the liver.

'Poor Dad drove to Melbourne and just turned up at each of our doors, unannounced, one evening. That was unusual, as Dad rarely came down by himself, so we knew something bad had happened. We didn't have time for coffee or small talk. He just told me straight that Mum had secondaries and that things didn't look good. He cried, I cried and then he left and was on his way to my sister and brother.'

That was already an exceedingly challenging and emotional time for Jodie. She was pregnant with her third child and her second had just turned one. 'I rang Mum, who, surprisingly, was okay. I was a mess. Mum told me she'd known for a couple of weeks and had now come to terms with the diagnosis. She hadn't wanted to tell us until she was sure,' explains Jodie.

'Mum was only six months short of what she felt was her five-year clearance, but she was pragmatic in playing the hand that she

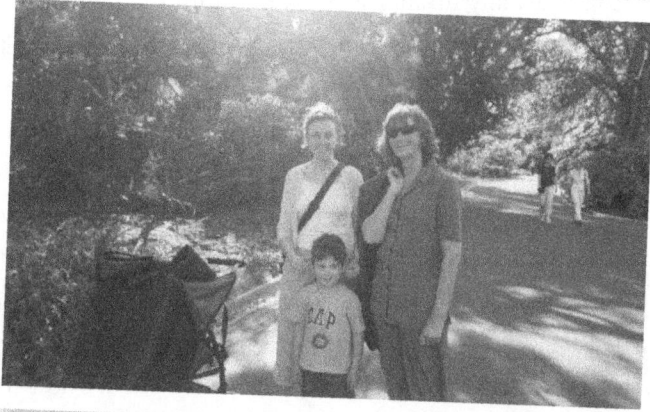

Jodie O'Keeffe and son, with Beverley Whitfield

was dealt. She knew there was no surgery that could help and she would face another brutal round of chemotherapy.

'She had been overextending herself; she was looking after her elderly father, back at school teaching and spending time with her grandchildren. She was trying to fit everything in.'

Beverley's new round of chemotherapy was powerful, often leaving her in hospital with low white cells and high temperatures. But it was effective, as her tumour markers were improving. Nevertheless, her body was struggling against the potent chemical onslaught and the dosage was continually cut back. Beverley's nails fell out and she regularly succumbed to bouts of viral and staph infections, but her only option was to endure.

By June 2004 Beverley finished her chemotherapy treatment and delighted in her newest grandson, Curtis. Life was good and Beverley and her family were positive about the future. However, after four months of joyous living, regular scans and tests showed the tumours in the liver continuing to grow, so further treatment was needed. An innovative new form of chemotherapy, Xeloda, was prescribed.

'Mum was relatively happy about this latest wonder drug for liver cancer because it could be taken in tablet form at home and she didn't have to spend more time in the oncology ward. An added bonus was that there was usually no hair loss. Sadly Mum seemed to get every side effect and with this drug the skin on her hands and feet peeled off, making it hard to walk.'

At this stage Jodie realised that things weren't going according to plan — her mother's reaction to the drug was quite severe. But she blocked out these personal concerns and, with her siblings, decided to maintain a positive outlook, especially around her mother.

'By Christmas Eve it was obvious to me and my sister, Linda, that the disease was probably terminal. Wrapping Christmas presents as a distraction, we vocalised our deepest fears. The hardest thing in dealing with Mum's cancer was to acknowledge she was dying. We kept asking ourselves if that meant we had given up. But we knew if we were facing this awful reality, then we needed to express our feelings to her while she was "fully" alive. This was really important for us. Mum and Dad weren't as open about it, but that was their way.

'We didn't know what was going to happen, but it was very important for Linda and I to tell Mum how much we loved her and to thank her for being such a wonderful mother. For me, it was a big thing to let her know, while she was alert and aware and able to take it in, that she was the best.'

Jodie sits in silence momentarily, sifting through her memories, and I notice tears glistening on her face. But she doesn't fight them.

'Christmas 2004 was special. We told Mum that we didn't know what the future held, but we were grateful for all she'd done for us. She took her headscarf off for the first time in months and she looked really good — although she was coughing a lot, was very tired and becoming increasingly frail.'

The chemotherapy was taking its toll, but Beverley continued taking the tablets as prescribed, suffering in silence.

'She kept taking them, no matter what damage the side effects caused. She ended up in hospital and the doctors decided to stop the treatment until she could regain some strength and shake off the worst of the side effects.'

Over the following days Beverley's severe reaction to the

treatment worsened, and she gradually stopped talking and eating and eventually lost consciousness. No one had expected such a rapid decline. Jodie and her family feared the worst. The doctors decided to treat her with steroids and antibiotics. When they took effect, Beverley woke up and was able to talk.

'We then realised Mum was angry. The holy grail of the new chemo that she had laid all her faith in had nearly killed her. She wasn't ready to go and she was totally annoyed. She had wanted to survive and the promise of the new drug didn't deliver,' Jodie says.

Though Beverley's condition improved for a while, it became increasingly obvious to everyone that she was dying. The family rallied and vowed that at least one of them would be by her side at all times — for however long Beverley had left.

'The month before she died was a time of emotional stress and intense pressure on us and our own families,' says Jodie. 'Our lives revolved around making Mum's last days as peaceful and loving as possible. It was also a time of coming to terms with our own personal loss.

'I was really pleased we had told Mum that we loved her at Christmas, because when you are losing someone, you don't have much time when they are actually awake and able to take it in.'

Beverley's friends came in to say their goodbyes. 'She knew she was dying and in her more lucid moments she'd check with us that she was still alive,' says Jodie. 'One day, out of the blue, she suggested I might help to choose the music for her funeral.'

But those moments of clarity became fewer, and by the start of February Beverley's husband, children and their families were emotionally and physically shattered. They were not coping well and wondered how long they could keep themselves positive.

Beverley died on 15 February 2005. 'We knew there was no longer any hope and so her death was in a way a release and a relief for us, and for her,' says Jodie.

Knowing Jodie from our days working together closely at the Commonwealth Games, the emotion with which she spoke these

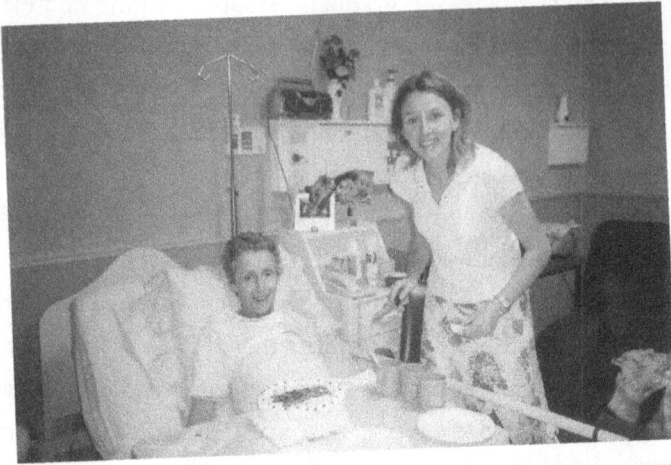

Beverley with Jodie

words touches me deeply. What I observe is the unbidden outpouring of grief of a thoughtful and loving daughter for her late mother, and it humbles me.

But the end of Beverley's life marked the start of a reconstruction of Jodie's life. She sought counselling to help her make sense of what had happened, so she could eventually turn her focus to the future.

'In 2005, with Kylie Minogue's diagnosis, breast cancer was everywhere — on TV, in newspapers and magazines. I was a little cynical at that time, because everyone was so upbeat and positive about Kylie recovering, but a lot of women die,' says Jodie.

'This is one of the reasons I wanted to tell Mum's story — not as a harbinger of death or to create fear, but just to acknowledge that some women do die from breast cancer. It is a terrible disease.

'It also seemed to me at that time that everything connected with breast cancer is focused on survival. There didn't seem to be much information about what might happen, about what we could expect if things didn't go well for Mum. We struggled and had to learn so much by ourselves about our journey towards Mum's death because there was just nothing out there, or we didn't know who to ask.'

While the grief of her mother's death is still palpable and raw, it isn't life-consuming and has not left Jodie fearful of her future or that of her daughter.

'I can only be optimistic for the future. Going round in my head is the reality that Mum got cancer and she died, and questions about why that happened to her have no answers, so I have to let it go. It has happened and I have to move on,' Jodie adds with a positive smile.

'Every six months I have tests; I self-examine regularly and I exercise and eat well to stay healthy, so if the worst happens I have the best chance of survival. The ultrasound tests and mammograms do bring a grave reality front and centre for me, although I don't go in thinking they will reveal any cancer. Being realistic, if I am going to get breast cancer, the best I can do is to find it as early as possible and then deal with it,' she says pragmatically.

'Seeing what's happened to Mum, I've got a renewed sense of life. She was 57 when she died. I'm 35 so if, because of my family history, I don't have a lot of time left then I want to make sure that I do as much with my life as possible. This is my life and I am living it now.'

Jodie's daughter, Ruby, now six, still finds her grandmother's death frightening and is often anxious that Jodie will die. 'I've made a deal with her that we will die together, which relieves her fears of being left behind. These are the conversations we can have now, because we have all gone through Mum's death.

'Before Mum died I had very little experience of death, and I am surprised how poorly our society deals with it. With hindsight and experience, I think we should talk about death more often as part of our life cycle, so we aren't as afraid to deal with it.

'And if we are faced with someone dying, we should acknowledge that and talk about their life. Celebrate who they are, what they have done, and let them know they've had an impact. It seems sad that we say these things at funerals — too late. Cancer gives us time and opportunity to say things when they are relevant and not have regrets later on,' she adds.

'We stayed in the hospital with Mum every day and night, and once she'd gone we took comfort in our efforts — we'd done our very best. It was a privilege for us to care for her in her last days. We didn't waste time in false hopes, but filled her life with love, dignity and respect right to the end.'

We stand up ready to go and embrace. Then Jodie leaves me with some parting words. 'Death isn't that bad. I can't stop it, so I just accept it. Meanwhile I have a life to live — to the full.'

Hello FOAM lovelies

This afternoon I have my final 'general radiation blast'.

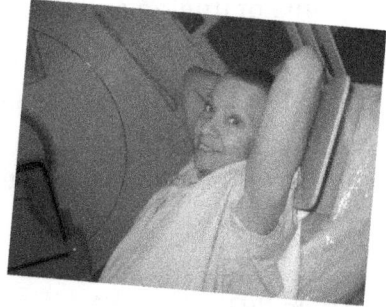

So after starting the planning and the treatment in early October, the time has finally arrived when I can see that the end is in sight. I will have had 30 total breast radiations, and tomorrow I start the final 5 spot radiations. These last five are high-dose radiation on the scar tissue surrounding the position where the tumour was, just so any tiny residue is totally zapped.

So **Wednesday December 3rd** will be a milestone for me — the end of my invasive insurance treatments against cancer.

219 days since I was diagnosed, 219 days of looking inwards at my health and my life, 219 days of being blessed by wonderful gifts and opportunities that may never have happened, 219 days of growing and learning and loving!

I move on to medicinal treatments soon, but next week is the last of my daily visits to the West Wing — and let me tell you, my West Wing has been far less exciting than the TV series of the same name.

I have also recently made several big lifestyle changes in my professional life so these coming weeks are a time of wonder for me!

December heralds the start of summer and this is my time. A time of fruition and blooming and blossoming after the growth of spring. After all my treatments I am now excited to begin this new phase of AnneMarie.

Thank you for helping me to this place ... and now we party!!!!!!!!!!!

Smile BIG.

AM

Helen Duroux's Journey

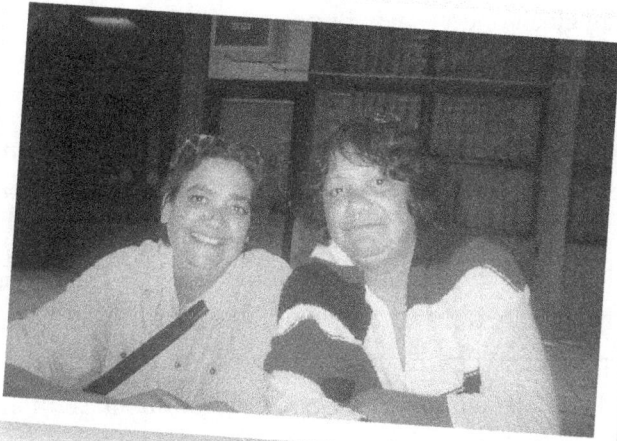

'I affirmed every day that I was a strong black woman and I could do anything if I decided to. And here I am now — still a strong black woman. I have got through so that I can continue the purpose I was meant to do — look after my Indigenous people.'

'The day I was diagnosed with breast cancer, my partner at the time freaked out, telling me most of his aunties had died of breast cancer and he thought that was the end of me, too. But no way was this disease going to kill me. I said to him, "Stop right there. I am a strong black woman and I will get through this!"'

This mantra — and the personal determination of Helen Duroux to not only get through this potentially fatal disease but also to use it as a life-changing catalyst — is inspirational.

As we sit and chat about her journey with breast cancer in a suburban coffee shop, I can't help but think that Helen's diagnosis has been a gift, albeit one she didn't want or wish for. For Helen, it was a timely reminder of her true purpose and passion in this life. And for her Aboriginal community, it was a godsend.

Helen was diagnosed seven years ago but she doesn't remember much about receiving the diagnosis and the subsequent events. 'It was all a complete blur and I don't really think about it any more. Until today, I didn't realise it was so long ago. Everything happened so quickly back then. I was drawn along into a type of whirlwind,' Helen explains.

She'd had a small lump in her breast for about 12 months but didn't do anything about it. 'I knew it was there but with all the unwanted stresses that were going on in my life at the time, it didn't seem that important.

'I gradually became more aware of it after moving to Queensland from Tenterfield, and more so after my auntie died from cancer. The lump was very small and it wasn't sore or painful, but as I was trying to sort out my life, I guess it just didn't get much attention,' she admits.

'I was doing a lot of work in the Indigenous community at Tenterfield back then, and that was the main trigger for moving north, as well as a break-up with the father of my four children. Welfare work is so draining. It becomes just too difficult to keep going on and on. I was elected onto the ATSIC board down in New South Wales, and in Tenterfield I was on the Local Aboriginal Land Council and the Aboriginal Community Housing Corporation board. As well,

I spent a lot of time — and devoted a great deal of personal energy — working with the young black kids.

'But I was a mother to my four children first of all, and all of the voluntary work started getting too hard to handle. I felt like I was carrying the whole community. I had always been involved with Indigenous affairs but it got to a point where it was too demanding. My marriage split up and so I sold everything and filled up the ute. My kids and I moved to Toowoomba and eventually ended up settling permanently in Brisbane.'

Looking back, Helen now recognises that she was totally burnt out and that the stress in her life had left her vulnerable to disease. Eventually she decided to have the lump in her breast investigated.

'Being new to Brisbane, I had no idea of where to go so I just went to the local doctor, who organised a mammogram for me. The results were suspicious so he said I needed further tests.'

She was booked in to see Dr Furnival, one of the highly respected oncology doctors at the Royal Brisbane Hospital, who somehow had a vacancy just when the receptionist called to get an appointment. After, in her words, 'lots of poking, prodding and examining', the doctor told her that the lump was malignant and it needed to be cut out immediately.

'I was rushed into surgery for a lumpectomy in the next two days. I didn't really ask any questions. This doctor was very well respected; he knew what was best for me and I trusted him. I didn't know my way around medical matters at all so I accepted what my doctor, who was the best in his business, advised me to do. However, everything happened so quickly and with so much urgency, that all I can really recall is that it was a busy blur for me.

'Fortunately the lump was very small — about the size of my fingernail — and only two nodes were infected. It was very scary. The fact that there were two nodes with cancer cells floating around in them made me very nervous about whether the cancer had completely gone or would eventually turn up somewhere else. Everyone assured me it was okay, but you can't help being a little worried, although I tried not to think about it too much,' Helen says.

A three-month program of chemotherapy was recommended, followed by radiation. Chemotherapy was to be a watershed for Helen.

'I was really sick for the first chemo session. But I worked out why. When I finished that first chemo treatment the nurse, who was very kind, told me to go home and to expect that I would feel very sick that night about 1am.

'And at exactly 1am I did feel awfully ill.

'The nurse had also told me that I would be nauseous and not able to do much for the next few days. And again I did feel off colour and couldn't do much at all. At first I thought to myself, "That nurse was right." But then I realised it was a self-fulfilling prophecy — the power of suggestion.

'I knew I didn't want it to be that way so the second time I went in for chemo, I decided that I wasn't going to accept being so debilitated, and I'd be more positive. By the third time I had convinced myself that I was going to be okay — and I was. In fact, my daughter came around to visit me the day after and I was out pottering in the garden. That was proof to me of the power of suggestion. So I was determined to suggest to myself that I would be fine — and I was.' She adds with a huge smile, 'And I still am today.

'I began reading everything positive I could. I really started believing in the power of positive thoughts. I read books like *Chicken Soup for the Soul*. I loved those books and they helped me so much. I did lots of meditation and continually reinforced my personal mantra. "I am a strong black woman and I can get through anything if I decide to,"' she says proudly.

'I have used that attitude to help me through lots of tough times in my past, including domestic violence and having to move around the country. But getting cancer was a big one, and I knew an optimistic mind-set would carry me through this battle.'

Losing her hair from the drugs was another time that saw the emergence of Helen as the 'strong black woman'.

'I remember I was sitting in the lounge with a cup of coffee a couple of weeks into treatment. I knew my hair was falling out because everywhere I'd move I'd leave trails of hair. But this day as I finished my coffee I looked into the bottom of the cup — and there was my hair. I told my partner, "It's time."

'He used clippers and shaved my head. I went to have a shower, but was crying so hard all I could do was sit in the shower. I sobbed for ages. People kept knocking on the bathroom door to see if I was alright. It was the hardest thing I've ever had to do. I coped with drains and tubes in my body; I managed to get through chemo and radiation — but losing my hair was the absolute worst. It hurt the most,' she confesses.

'The day I was having the lumpectomy, my brother rang me and asked me if the doctors were cutting my breast off. I told him that they would be taking some of my breast, but as far as I was concerned they could cut them both off if it meant living longer. I dealt with that much better than losing my hair,' she says.

Helen decided to wear what she describes as mad scarves and hats. 'Being so devastated when I lost my hair meant that I was very excited when it started growing back. Lots of the ladies I was having treatment with told me that my hair may grow back grey, blonde or even red. I told them I wouldn't mind being blonde. Of course, it grew back very dark but in the tightest ringlets you've ever seen. I thought that was hilarious because in my youth I'd paid what was a small fortune for me back then to have perms and look just as I did now!'

She laughs as she recalls how, when her uncle came to visit, he wouldn't believe that the luxurious ringlets were natural.

Helen is a Murri woman from the Kamilaroi mob and is intensely proud of her cultural heritage. Being a strong black woman is the core of her existence. 'Because of my Aboriginality, I have always drawn strength from it and I get a lot of power from that. I have enormous respect for so many of the Aboriginal women who have lived hard lives, but have overcome the difficulties to be leaders in not only our Indigenous communities but, for many of them, our country.

'I've always admired those Aboriginal women and drawn inspiration from their experiences. I think that if they can do it, then so can I. And I take that positive personal power into every day of my life. That personal strength was especially important during my battle with cancer.'

When I ask Helen whether, in her view, Aboriginal people experience illness, disease and treatment in culturally specific ways, she shakes her head. Although she points out that for Aboriginal women, the importance of women's groups is very powerful, she sees no real differences. 'When I was going through cancer, it was very personal, but because I didn't really know anyone in Brisbane I did feel quite alone. In the last few years I have got together with a Murri women's group in Redcliffe. They are amazingly supportive, and until I joined that group, I didn't realise how important these women were in my life. They would have been wonderful during my cancer journey. Now I try to be as supportive of women with cancer as I can.

'During my illness, my family would ring and be supportive, but essentially my children and I were on our own. So to keep my spirits up I wrote in a journal every day. Any quote I'd see from books I'd been reading — affirmations or things people said — went in there. I sometimes pull it out now and re-read it. I am proud of how strong I stayed.'

Like most women, Helen didn't know much about the nature of breast cancer and it hadn't really touched her closely. 'I lost my grandfather to cancer and one of my aunties also had cancer. She died of uterine cancer, but I think she may have had breast cancer initially. She didn't want surgery, but I found out later that had she had the hysterectomy that doctors advised her to have, she would have survived. That memory stuck in my mind when I started noticing the lump in my breast. I think it was the memory of my Auntie Val dying that really spurred me to investigate my lump.'

When I ask Helen why she thinks she got breast cancer she answers, 'Quite simply, I blame stress.

'While I am certain that stress was the main reason I got cancer,

I can't help but wonder if my past workplaces also aggravated the tumour's growth. I worked in orchards, cotton fields and tobacco farms where DDT and chemicals were sprayed.

'But the constant tensions, strains and anxiety in my life were certainly the root cause of it. That was the reason, too, that I had to move up to Queensland. So when I got cancer, I was determined that I would adjust my life. I did lots of meditation, breathing, reading and just focusing on relaxing. I loved to potter around in my garden and I often sat at the waterfront just being quiet. I also maintained a very healthy diet. I think the fact I have always eaten fresh fruit and vegetables helped me fight the disease.'

Helen is deeply spiritual. To me, it seems that she draws strength from a variety of spiritual traditions and practices. 'Part of my Aboriginality gives me a spiritual awareness that is getting stronger as I grow older. So I also would focus on bringing light into my breast, imagining healing and then sending the light out with the impurities. I had to let the bad things go,' she says.

'The cancer really made me look at what was important. I had a life to live and there was no way I was going under again. So I eliminated stress. I broke up with my partner and I am not anywhere as obsessive about having a perfectly tidy house. I am on my own, taking it a bit easy and really loving my life.'

Helen does, however, acknowledge that in prioritising what is important to her, she recognises her mission is to help her Indigenous community — in particular, the youth. Today she runs training programs on literacy and numeracy and referral services.

'The funny thing is I am back doing all the things that brought on the stress in the first place. But this time I have a second chance to do it knowingly and manage it. I've learned my lesson about stress and I won't let the pressure get to me again. I also know that this is what I am meant to do in this life.

'I am good at what I do and I have to stop trying to help absolutely everyone, because I know I can't stretch myself too far. I do the best I can to help as many people as I can.

'I know education is the saviour for these young people. The satisfaction in seeing young Indigenous people getting jobs and apprenticeships is fantastic. One of the girls in my program recently came back and urged me to keep the programs going because "You got me back on track and I want you to do the same for my younger sister." That moment I just knew I was doing the right thing!'

Although Helen refers to her work in a low-key, self-deprecating way, I suspect that she finds it extremely fulfilling. But its importance to her doesn't stop there.

'My work in the Aboriginal community is probably the only reason I got through the cancer and lived. I hadn't finished what I was supposed to do! My community work is now not a load to carry but a blessing. I believe everyone is worth saving and I love seeing the positive changes in young people.'

Helen has a strong belief that her life is not completely random, that she has a purpose. She tells me she is 'dragged around by old black spirits. They tell me that I am meant to be here doing what I am doing and I always tend to be in the right place at the right time. I feel tied to that black spirituality and the older I get, the more power — power in the sense of fulfilling desires for my people — I feel coming to me.'

Helen tells the story from many years ago of when she and her mother were walking in the bush, doing an inspection for ATSIC. Her mother and she followed the men, winding up through a rocky outcrop. Halfway up the hill Helen felt paralysed and slumped to the ground, unable to move in spite of her mother urging her to get up. Her mother went to the rock wall behind them, put her hands on the rock and spoke in a strange language. Then she returned, telling Helen to get up and walk. Helen stood up easily and was able to walk again. She wanted to know what had happened. Helen's mother told her that she had 'talked to the spirits of the old people, and told them to let you pass because you belong to me'.

From that time, Helen knew that the black spirits within were an integral part of who she was and is today. She knew that in challenging times — like during her battle with cancer — she could call on her black spirits.

'I was educated in the Christian system and so I do have a faith, but I've always personally believed that the Aboriginal spirituality is as strong as that. I always tell people there is a greater power, but it is up to each of us in what we believe.

'Right from the beginning of this journey with breast cancer I was determined to get through. I affirmed every day that I was a strong black woman and I could do anything if I decided to. And here I am now — still a strong black woman. I have got through so that I can continue the purpose I was meant to do — look after my Indigenous people; help and encourage them to get an education and therefore a chance at a good life.'

Yes. That's Helen Duroux — the strong black woman!

From: AnneMarie
Subject: FINALLY — FREE AT LAST
Sent: 4 December 2003

Hello FOAMs

Yesterday at 4.26pm the radiation light finished beaming protection onto my right breast.

I dressed and walked out of Level 3 in the Oncology Section of the hospital, knowing that at this moment I am cancer-free. As I walked to the car, I reflected on the millions of minutes I had spent preparing for this moment, dreaming of the end of treatments. Free at last ...

Although I have always felt over the past 219 days that the cancer 'organised' my diary, I never felt cancer dominated my soul or spirit. So in a sense the end of treatments just gives me more time for the family, the friends and the fun of living my life to the max!

I know this is not the end of my journey — that will stay with me in many different and exciting forms as I grow towards the wonderfully disgraceful 94-year-old woman in the purple hat. I look forward to sharing many a champers in the following 40-something years!!

Next year I intend having a FOAMy party to celebrate and look forward to clinking glasses with each and every one of you to say thank you for your support in the myriad of ways it has been delivered — and always with love.

But first I have to recover my health and energy so that I can actually stay awake after 8pm at night!

Thank you, FOAMs.

Keep on smiling

AM

Meredith Campbell's Journey

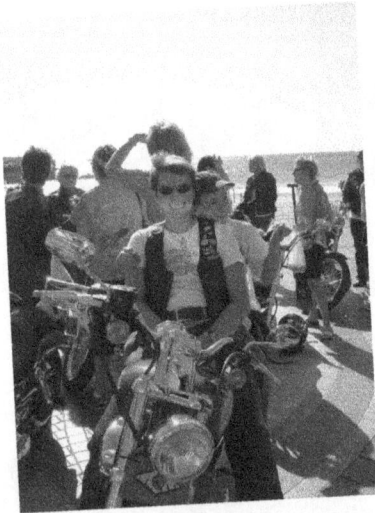

'I asked myself why. "Why was I doing all this?" "Why was I working so hard?" The first year after breast cancer is always challenging and confronting, and I was starting to question where I was going and was it worth it?'

What if breast cancer is just the start of an incredible journey?

For Meredith Campbell, being diagnosed with breast cancer has given her the ride of her life — literally. It was the trigger for what has become an amazing story.

Meredith and fellow breast cancer survivor Megan Dwyer created Amazon Heart, an international organisation that celebrates life for survivors of breast cancer and at the same time changes the world through advocacy, fundraising and local community projects.

Before being diagnosed with breast cancer in 2000, Meredith had been involved with a variety of not-for-profit charities and had worked at the Cancer Council for a number of years. Consequently, she was aware of breast cancer and its impact on our society but had never imagined it would touch her so directly.

'I found it very personally challenging to go from working for a cause to actually being a part of that cause. It was a big psychological adjustment for me and even more so as a young woman. I never expected to have to confront dangers to my health, face my mortality or to question my view of the future at this age,' she says.

At 33 years old, Meredith was an international sailor and recognised around the world as a respected marketing professional. 'I was fit and healthy, had a six-year-old son and, with no family history, breast cancer was the last thing I had thought would happen to me. It made no sense to me at all.'

It wasn't until 18 months after her cancer diagnosis, on a charity walk in the USA, that Meredith found a deeper meaning to life — one that sent her in a totally new direction.

'I'd gone to America to participate in the Avon Walk for Breast Cancer. Over 3000 women walk 100 kilometres in three days, and it is a spectacularly successful fundraising event. At the time, I was working with Kids Help Line and I went over to look at the Avon concept, thinking that by participating in it I could see if the principle could be adapted and brought back here to Brisbane.

'I went with a little trepidation and lined up at five in the morning with all the other women — with no personal disclosure that I, too, was a cancer survivor, only admitting to working for a charity in Australia. On the starting line I was introduced to a young woman who told me she had had breast cancer and, without thinking, I blurted out, "Me, too — you look so good." I always struggled with breast cancer being a part of my identity and even for this event I had left my "Survivor" shirt and hat back in my bags — not really wanting to own up to it,' she admits.

She did eventually wear the 'Survivor' shirt and found that it did bring an unexpected bond and connection with those other people who'd gone through a similar journey. 'I'd be standing at traffic lights, and in the 30 seconds they took to change to green, many women would come up and tell me I looked great or encourage me to stay strong. It felt good.

'This event started to make some sense of my diagnosis. I found myself no longer denying that I had had breast cancer but able to own it and accept that cancer was part of who I was — but it certainly was not my identity,' Meredith explains. 'And this was probably what led me to the path of Amazon Heart.'

Meredith admits that the first time she talked with the media about her personal story and the founding of Amazon Heart she was very emotional and found it extremely difficult. 'But,' she says, 'the more you tell your cancer story, the less power it has over you. Amazon Heart became a part of my history and this is how I have dealt with being a young woman diagnosed with breast cancer.'

Meredith remembers the exact moment she was told she had cancer. It was 10am on 28 September 2000 and she was at home watching Jenny Armstrong and Belinda Stowell win Australia's first ever Olympic gold medal in sailing. 'I had raced in the 470s class, which is the one the girls raced, and so I was glued to the television when the phone rang. It was my doctor telling me that I had breast cancer. To say I was shocked is an understatement.

'I had been to see him after finding a lump in my breast. So I had the screening mammogram and the fine-needle biopsy and I stayed home from work the following day to wait for the results — and of course to watch Jenny and Belinda sail their final race. I was expecting the lump was a cyst — certainly nothing serious,' she says.

'Hearing the bad news was one of those moments of raw human emotion that strips you bare. Here I was in the middle of an ecstatic moment with the girls winning gold at the Olympic Games in Sydney and I'm in my loungeroom in Brisbane being told I have breast cancer. Once reality stepped in, I was in a whirlwind doing all those things you need to organise, like calling my boss and finding a surgeon. I was thrown into the middle of a surreal world.'

Meredith was diagnosed with a Stage 2 Grade 3 tumour and large node involvement. 'In fact I had a larger tumour in my lymph nodes than in my breast, so this was serious. I realised this was an acute diagnosis.

'However, I also knew there are no guarantees in life and we just have to deal with what we have,' Meredith philosophically reminds me.

She then tells me about a quote from the *Lord of the Rings* film that sustained her through this challenge. 'In the first movie, there is a scene where the troop is going through the mines of Moria. It is dark and it's scary, and Frodo is sitting there saying he wished this had never happened and that the Ring had never come to him. He didn't want to deal with it. And Gandalf says to him, "Well, that's what everyone says in a situation like this; but that's not the choice you get to make. The choice is what you will do with the time you were given."

'For me, I didn't choose to get breast cancer, and of course no one chooses to get cancer. I can't change the fact I did, and so the choice for me was what would I do with the time I had? What would I do with each day that lay ahead of me?'

Once diagnosed, Meredith then made her choices. She had a lumpectomy and an auxillary dissection. That was followed by a three-month course of Epirubicin chemotherapy, then three months of radiation treatment. She finished the regime with three more months of chemotherapy, this time using Taxol.

'So that pretty much wiped me out for most of a year. I was pretty angry having to go through chemo, but I psyched myself up to see it as a challenge. The whole nature of the treatment was quite depressing, especially as a young woman,' she says. 'I'd go in and be the youngest person in the room. I'd look around and think that I didn't belong there.'

She tolerated the chemo quite well and the only time she felt nauseous or unwell was during the final treatment of the first round of treatments. 'I think that was a psychological purging. I got home and hurled my guts out and shouted "That's done!"

'During that time, I went through a phase of eating lots of McDonald's food, which didn't help with my weight gain, but it made me happy,' she laughs.

'Radiation gave me a little physical break as it wasn't so taxing on my body. It also gave my hair a chance to start growing back—although it was very dark and afro-style curls, which was kind of freaky. But then it all fell out again when I had the second round of treatments. By the time I'd finished the second three months of chemotherapy, I had no hair or eyebrows or eyelashes. It's a bad look — you can get away with having no hair and just looking a bit butch, but without the eyelashes and eyebrow it is just bizarre.'

Meredith chuckles as she recalls that the second time her hair returned, it was totally grey, 'So I quickly dyed it and I have absolutely no idea what colour it is now. When your hair grows back it is just like a foreign object. I suddenly had curls where I had always had straight hair,' she says with a shake of her now auburn waves.

All the way through her treatments Meredith had felt that she just needed to get through each day. When they were all finished, she decided that her life would go back to what it was. Because it was important to her to maintain normality in her life, she worked most of the time during the medication period.

Just before her diagnosis, Meredith had been asked to go overseas as a guest speaker at an international conference. She was then to travel to India as part of her job with a not-for-profit organisation. That had been put on hold. 'But as soon as I had done with the medical whirlwind, I was desperate to reclaim my life,' she says.

'So six weeks after treatments I went to India — a country that can transform you. I thought I'd had a very difficult year but I wasn't really prepared for the shock of going out to the remote villages. The people lived in abject poverty, but I was astonished that they lived their lives with such hope and joy. They were full of life with no despair. They were looking for something better in their lives, but not miserable at all. Every day they were just trying to make the best of their situation. I had never been into such a poor place that had no self-pity. It actually transformed me and helped me to realise that there are certainly worse things you can go through than breast cancer. It really picked me up,' she acknowledges humbly.

Returning from India, Meredith threw herself back into her career. 'I've always been a dedicated worker and was very successful. But I then had an epiphany moment. I asked myself why. "Why was I doing all this?" "Why was I working so hard?" The first year after breast cancer is always challenging and confronting, and I was starting to question where I was going and was it worth it?' she says.

'After the Avon walk, I had put my body under a lot of stress — walking over 100 kilometres on hard pavements in intense heat over three days was tough, and I collapsed the arch in my right foot. It was an agonising pain, like a knife was being driven into it. Now — as anyone who has been diagnosed with cancer will tell you — as soon as you get a sore area, you immediately think, "Bone cancer, and this is it!"'

With lots of external stresses also happening at this time, Meredith put off seeing a doctor for two months, 'in case it was bad news'. Finally she decided to go. 'I thought that all the stress I was creating was certainly not good for my health and I reasoned that if the news was bad and the damn thing had come back, maybe I would look back and wonder what I had been doing with my life. Luckily, it turned out to be a physical injury, which healed fine, but that conversation with myself had far-reaching effects. I asked myself if this is the way I really wanted to live my life and would I have regrets?'

The answer to that soul-searching question was yes: she would have regrets. Armed with this self-knowledge, Meredith knew that nothing less than a fulfilling and purposeful life was acceptable to her, so she resigned from her job and decided to work as a consultant. This would give her far more flexibility with her time and allow her to discover her life direction.

That weekend after her resignation, in 2002, she went to Sydney to compete in the sailing regatta at the Gay Games. 'I was watching the American sailing team walking around, all smug and confident, when I noticed one of the women was bald and had temporary tattoos covering her head. My teammates were joking about the "scary Americans", but I saw that she had no eyebrows or eyelashes and I immediately recognised a woman on chemo,' she says.

'When I was bald I stood out, and I found it difficult wherever I was, be it at work, at the supermarket or just walking around the street. People found the need to come up to me and tell me all of their most gruesome stories about cancer. They were often very intrusive, asking questions about what I had and what was wrong with me. And I've noticed, with these strangers, that everyone dies in their world. Thank you for sharing that as I sit with my six-year-old son! So on seeing this woman at sailing, I was understanding of her privacy and didn't want to pry,' says Meredith of her initial meeting with Megan Dwyer.

'About halfway through the regatta, I happened to be sitting beside Megan and we started chatting. It came up that she had breast cancer. We found we had shared similar experiences as young women battling breast cancer, so by the end of the competition Megan and I had become very good friends.'

Megan returned to California but Meredith and she kept in touch via email and telephone. 'She was the first young woman who I had met with breast cancer, and it was wonderful to be able to share some of our many common interests. We also had similar attitudes. We both knew we wanted to get back into an active life. Megan was only five weeks out of chemo when she did a triathlon. Now that is one gutsy woman!'

But getting on with things was how both Meredith and Megan approached their life post-cancer. 'You almost feel superhuman. You want to do everything. I went to India in searing heat. What was I going to do? Sit at home and feel miserable? Of course not. My life is a work in progress and I was trying to make sense of who I was and who I will be,' Meredith explains.

'After the very lengthy email exchanges about what it is really like to be young and have breast cancer, and how we got through it all — especially as it had taken so long for us to find someone who really understood how we were feeling — Megan and I thought that it may be useful for other women to read about our journey. So we decided to collaborate and write and publish a book about our journey.

'It was very cathartic for us to produce the book *Amazon Heart — Coping with Breast Cancer Warrior Princess Style*. It is very warts and all and has been quite successful. What is more important to us is that we've had lots of women tell us that it helped them.'

After producing the book, Meredith and Megan wondered what they could do next. Meredith had always looked for opportunities to live her life fully and after returning from India she'd got her motorcycle licence. 'Don't really know why. I had always been a responsible mother and very professional in my career; it was just one of those things I wanted to do before I was 40,' she says lightly. Megan was then inspired to follow suit, also getting her licence.

'We were then talking about ways to launch and promote the book. I'd heard of a group called the Fenceliners, who several years earlier had done an adventurous motorcycle ride around Australia with a couple of breast cancer survivors. They also did a paddle down the Murray and a bicycle ride around Tasmania. In fact, I was a little annoyed that they'd done their motorcycle ride before I was diagnosed,' she chuckles.

Meredith thought it was a great idea, but these were older women who could afford to take lots of time to enjoy their escapades, whilst she knew that most younger women didn't have that luxury of time off from work and family.

'So Megan and I planned to do a one-week bike ride in California, America, from San Diego up to San Francisco. And we decided to find a motorcycle company to give us the bikes!' she says.

'I went off to the States and we made a few calls — hoping! Then one day we got a call from Harley Davidson in Milwaukee, who said they loved our idea. So we jumped onto a plane and met with them. They were incredibly generous right upfront. They agreed to lend us 20 brand-new motorcycles and truck them to and from the start and finish of the ride. They would provide leather jackets for all riders and even offered mechanical support along the way. They were just fantastic.'

In October 2004, with five Australian riders and 15 Americans, the dream of an adventure became a reality for the two women. They knew that the ride would be high profile, attract attention and therefore raise a lot of money. What they didn't anticipate was the personal and emotional impact it would have on those women who took part.

'At the end of the ride, all of the women were on a high. They said that for the first time they believed in themselves and their ability to build a new life after cancer. And then they asked where they were going next year.'

Amazingly, by Christmas the following year Harley Davidson had supported adventures in not only the USA but also in Australia and the United Kingdom. Amazon Heart Adventures had been born and was thriving. Buoyed by this success, Meredith and Megan expanded their vision as they contemplated what else they could do to empower breast cancer survivors.

'I thought back to my times in India and I wondered if we could take breast cancer survivors into Third World countries and undertake some community building projects. Megan and I also thought about trekking adventures. So the whole Amazon Heart thing just exploded.'

I get a sense of the adrenaline surge Meredith has experienced in the course of all this expansion. From time to time she shakes her head slightly, as if even she can't believe herself how quickly the enterprise took off.

The choice of the name and identity for these projects was the result of deep deliberation on the underpinning reason for establishing these adventures. 'It had been very difficult for me as a young woman with breast cancer to find positivity and connection with similar-minded women. I realised that at the heart of my experience was an emotional vulnerability which meant I cried quicker than before, or felt exposed to weaknesses or deep feelings more than ever before. Trying to reconcile that more vulnerable person with the independent woman I had been before cancer was a big challenge for me,' she explains.

'The name Amazon Heart reflected that personal exploration. *Amazon* represented the strong, empowered woman, and *Heart* was the emotional vulnerability that the breast cancer had brought. There is, of course, the ancient myth about Amazon women chopping off their right breast in order to fire their arrows more efficiently in war. So this name resonated strongly with our ideals.'

The title also sat well in the public arena, with Meredith receiving many emails from women who identified with the name telling her that they, too, were Amazon Warriors. 'In fact, 20 women that we know of have tattooed the Amazon Heart logo onto their bodies! Now that means they have truly adopted our vision,' she says with pride.

'Amazon Heart symbolised transformation — giving women power over their cancer experience. I had initially thought that Amazon Heart would be a one-off ride, but it exploded overnight. It is an incorporated charity in Australia, America and the UK, with independent boards. But the reality is that everything comes back to Megan and I, and we just can't keep doing it for ever. We need to keep our day jobs, and that's not possible given the amount of effort we both continue to put into Amazon Heart.'

'It literally takes all of our time after work and on weekends. I never wanted to be a huge conglomerate charity. I wanted it to be something that Megan and I did for the love of the cause, and did really well. I am passionate about the idea and very willing to share our experience and ideas because the benefits to participants are so valuable.

'A research project, conducted by the University of Queensland and the Cancer Council, validated that for women who participated in our adventures and projects, there was a measurable positive impact that our adventures had on their outlook for the future after breast cancer. Peer support isn't often externally validated, so this was rare and a very important finding. Indeed, it was such an exciting conclusion that Megan and I were invited to Washington to present at the World Cancer Congress and then at the UICC International Reach to Recovery Conference in Stockholm. In 2007, we also addressed the International Conference on Survivorship and Supportive Care in Cancer in Kuala Lumpur. That is a very rewarding acknowledgment for what we have done.'

Since the positive psychosocial impact of these adventures has been officially endorsed, Meredith's ideas have been taken up around the world, with rides now taking place through South Africa and Malaysia.

At the time of our interview, Megan and Meredith are working with the Cancer Council Queensland to formulate a 'how to' kit based on Amazon Heart Adventures and providing the tools and logistics to get these programs up and running anywhere in the world.

Whilst taking the ideas internationally will be a wonderful legacy, the truth is that Amazon Heart is really Megan and Meredith. When they step down, will this be the end of Amazon Heart Adventures?

'We know that we can impart so much knowledge and share our ideas with anyone who wants to replicate what we have done. But because so much of our DNA is embedded in each adventure or project, I know that Amazon Heart is really us. The exciting thing is that the concept will flourish and spread throughout the world — but we won't be running them. And that is okay,' Meredith says.

'They will be successful and valuable for those who participate, and that is a wonderful feeling — knowing our ideas have rippled through the world for good.

'This year, 2009 will be the final year. Two last rides — we think. Working full-time, I just can't keep taking time off to run these adventures. I never say never, and perhaps we may just cut back and do fewer projects, or we may collaborate with a larger organisation that can support our administration and organisation. Don't know — we'll just have to see.

'One of the other considerations that is probably camouflaged is that Amazon Heart Adventures takes a huge emotional toll on me, and on Megan. Because many of our participants have secondary cancer and are travelling with us to make every day of their lives count, we become very close. Unfortunately, from each trip, several of these women die. Having lost 15 friends in the past few years, the emotional toll — for me as a survivor — is very hard,' Meredith says sadly.

Reflecting on the past eight years, Meredith appreciates that since being diagnosed with the deadly disease, her life has definitely changed. 'I have grown in these past years, but I certainly wish there could have been a better way to personal development than getting breast cancer. But I am grateful that it caused me to re-evaluate a lot of things in my life. The experiences I've had — especially after forming Amazon Heart — have been amazing, both the bike rides and the active charity work in India.

'To work in places like India, returning each year to the village we work in and seeing the orphanages for AIDS victims we've built and the changes we have made in the quality of their life is very humbling,' she adds.

'Riding bikes around the world with amazing women on inspiring trips and at the same time raising over US$650,000 for charity also gives me a sense of pride and achievement.

'But when I look back and reflect on what has been most rewarding for me, it is the legacy of hope for women diagnosed with breast cancer. It is that inner transformation that Amazon Heart has been able to create in the lives of over 200 women who have participated in our journeys. That makes me feel really good.

'Amazon Heart changed the direction of my life. I've grown enormously as a woman. But breast cancer is a journey. It doesn't end — it is there for the rest of my life. But because of research and greater awareness, more and more women are enjoying life after breast cancer, and there is a greater focus on survivorship. More and more women are choosing how to live their lives in an active and positive manner after cancer,' she says. 'That's why Amazon Heart filled such an important niche.'

Perhaps the final word on Meredith's journey comes from her son, Dexter, who was only six years old when Meredith was diagnosed in 2000. He has always been very supportive of his mum and everything she does.

'Recently, Dexter had to do a school project on the most inspirational person in the world. He did it on me. That's when you know you've done something worthwhile,' she says, beaming with pride.

Amazon Heart was indeed the start of an incredible journey for Meredith Campbell — but, more importantly, the start of an incredible journey of hope and inspiration for the thousands of women with Amazon hearts throughout the world.

From: AnneMarie
Subject: CHRISTMAS THANK YOU
Sent: 15 December 2003

Dear FOAM Friends ...

As Christmas approaches very quickly I would like to thank
each of you for your wonderful support this year.

- True Friendship is like good health: *the true value of it is seldom known until it is lost.*
- Friends are difficult to find, hard to leave and impossible to forget.

I have been so blessed to have had such a wonderful group
of friends:

who listened when I was upset,
who celebrated when I was excited,
who loved when I was scared,
who gave advice when I was uncertain,
who inspired when I was doubtful,
but most of all,
who carried me through my challenging year,
allowing me to make it through
with Happiness and Courage on my shoulders.

On Friday I have my final surgery — to retrieve my port-
o-cath. It was suggested I leave it in place for the next
12 months — in case I need it. I won't and I want to draw
a line in the sands of my life as the end of treatments and
the beginning of my new life. It also allows me to have the

most wonderful Christmas present of all — a healthy, happy Christmas with family and an exciting new start in 2004.

Thank you, special FOAM friends, thank you for this year, and I wish each of you true peace and joy for the next year.

Starry smiles

AnneMarie

Susan Duncan's Journey

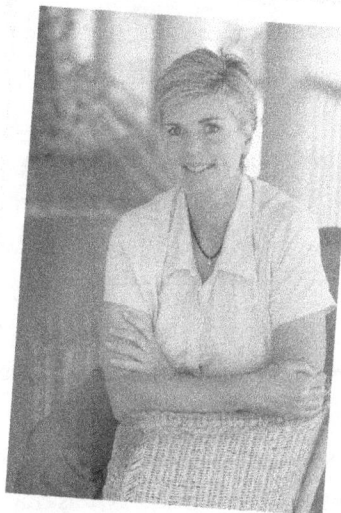

'I am conscious that every day must be cherished. I try never to do anything that I don't want to do. I try not to waste a single second of my life. I've had a wobble or two but I am content in whatever space I am in — living in the moment is instinctive now.'

everal years ago, as I battled my own breast cancer demons, I bought a book because I liked the sound of the title — *Salvation Creek, an Unexpected Life*. A year of intense treatments had bludgeoned irreparably what I thought of as my indomitable spirit. I knew nothing of the author or what the book was about, but the joyful idea of finding not only 'salvation' but an 'unexpected life' seemed to be the tonic I needed.

I read the book voraciously, even taking it with me to the loo. Then, as I almost finished page 154, I read the words, 'I felt a lump in my right breast.' Susan Duncan, the author, then goes on to describe, in the most compelling and honest manner, how she got herself through breast cancer. How she survived.

I remember at the time tearing through the pages and recognising our similar experiences. Little did I know at that time that we would also have in common the grief following the death of a much-loved spouse.

Now here I was at 'Tarrangaua', Susan's Pittwater paradise, sipping tea and devouring one of her now famous lemon cakes as she retold the story of her journey with breast cancer.

Susan admits that she knew very little about breast cancer before she discovered her lump. 'All I really knew was that it was something I didn't want to have. When I first began working at *The Australian Women's Weekly* when I was in my early 30s, there was a woman working with me who got breast cancer and died. I have a distinct and haunting memory of her in the bathroom at work, adjusting her wig and looking very grey. It scared me. She had the look of someone who was dying.'

Before her diagnosis in 1999, Susan confesses that her life was fairly self-destructive. 'My husband, Paul, and brother, John, had died several years earlier. At the time I'd put on the high heels and gone back to work quite quickly, until 18 months later I just collapsed, emotionally and physically. I quit my job at *New Idea*, sold my house and began the frightening job of reconfiguring my life without the two people who had always been the lynchpins.

'In the following few years, I drank like a fish, moved into inappropriate relationships and too often just moved from day to day in a blur. I don't know why: it was a form of insanity. I was another person. I suspect grief sent me mad for a while,' Susan bluntly admits.

There was no family history of breast cancer, although Susan tells me she 'certainly knew about cancer in the family. My husband died of a brain tumour, and my brother of the rare thymoma, so I knew that people die of cancer. I just didn't expect I would get it. But then none of us does, do we?

'I remember one day, several months before I was diagnosed. I was totally exhausted after doing a travel story on the luxury ocean liner *Queen Elizabeth II*. I hadn't eaten or drunk anything all day; and when I got home to the brown house where I was living at the time, I was so tired I didn't bother turning on any lights. I was in an emotional turmoil over my chaotic and shockingly desperate love life and I just crashed into bed without even bothering to turn on the lights. I remember thinking, "This is the sort of self-punishing behaviour that could trigger cancer." Looking back, perhaps I had a kind of sixth sense. Not long after, I felt a lump in my right breast and I knew I had to get it checked out.'

I saw the local doctor the following day, and he couldn't find anything but insisted that I have a mammogram. I was almost certain there was nothing seriously wrong. A cyst at the worst. So I felt pretty confident — or perhaps it was a case of denial — when I was examined at the clinic around the corner.'

Even when the nurse at the clinic asked to do a second mammogram on just her right breast, Susan believed it was only 'because it was a little blurry'. Expecting the all-clear, she didn't bother making another appointment with the doctor for the results. The receptionist rang two days later and insisted Susan come in 'sooner rather than later — Doctor will explain'.

'The next day "Doctor" gave me the bad news and, as I always do when I don't think I'll cope with what's happening, I escaped to my own imaginary, beautiful place and hoped that the worst wouldn't happen. If I didn't think about something bad, then of course it wouldn't happen,' she says.

Susan then went to a breast cancer specialist in Sydney and had the painful long-needle biopsy.

'As I waited for the results, I looked at the other anxious women in the waiting room and knew fear. I remembered being with my brother, John, as he went through an horrendous time with chemo, so I had laid out the ground rules with the specialist a week earlier when I had made my appointment. "If things are bad, I'm not having chemo, and," I added flippantly, "I'd rather buy a ticket to Italy and sit out death with great food, good wine and Dean Martin belting out 'Volare' on a bad sound system,"' explains Susan.

'So when I went back to get my results I sat down, looked at him and asked, "Do I buy a ticket to Italy?" He was very quiet and then slowly opened the file, his eyes intently focused on the written words. "Yep," he said, "it's Italy."

'Immediately I thought that meant I was going to die,' she adds. 'I shut down at that moment and again went into denial mode. I didn't want to know how advanced the cancer was or any other gory details. But I did hear that the tumour was right underneath the nipple and that my breast couldn't be saved. Again I retorted glibly, "Oh, well, I have two!"'

The doctor explained to Susan that she would need to have a mastectomy and that her lymph nodes would be removed (note: I was operated on just a few months before the technology changed) and tested to see if the malignancy had spread.

'I was very adamant that I wouldn't do chemo,' Susan says, but the doctor told her to hold back from any decisions until after surgery. No one could guess the prognosis until after surgery.

'Denial became my form of attack. Probably because I was too damned scared to ask about the extent of the disease. Or maybe I thought I could just ignore all the facts and deal with this in my own idiosyncratic way,' she says.

'As it turned out, my prognosis was not the best, but it was the second best. At the time, I thought that was pretty good and certainly better than no scenario at all. So I just got on with it.'

The tumour was the size of a pea and had been there a long time. But there was no way of removing the tumour carefully as it was directly under Susan's nipple. There was only a minute trace of the cancer in one lymph node.

While Susan now knew the facts, she still wanted to avoid chemotherapy. Her surgeon felt she could take that option but insisted she take Tamoxifen tablets for the next five years.

'I was relieved at his advice. I had seen the ravages of successively more potent chemo sessions when my brother was ill and I'd vowed I would never do it if I were in a similar situation. But that was then, and now I was facing my own mortality and I didn't really know what to do,' says Susan. 'So I went away to think about it.'

A little while later, after discussions with friends and colleagues, she decided to make an appointment with an oncologist to get a second opinion of her options.

'When I asked her what she would do if she was in my place, she told me she'd have the treatment because I had two types of cancer cells and one was a risk for me. That was enough. I really wanted to believe that having the four doses of chemo would guarantee I'd beat the disease. So I decided to go through with it, knowing that I would then have no regrets that I didn't do the hard yards when I should have,' she says pragmatically. 'But, mostly, I wanted the comfort of knowing that if cancer returned, I had done everything I could to beat it.'

Susan admits she nearly chickened out on the first treatment of chemo. 'I was walking round Royal North Shore Hospital and couldn't find the chemo treatment room. I thought that this was an omen telling me not to have the treatments. Then when I finally found my way and asked the nurse for reassurance that I was doing the right thing, she told me she'd have chemo if she had my kind of cancer. So I did the hard stuff, hoping that there wouldn't be any more in the future.'

After that first treatment Susan woke up in the middle of that night drenched in sweat. 'I think I went instantly into menopause,' she says. 'I showered and went back to bed but I was still burning up and it was the middle of winter. The next morning I felt fine and I got up and went to work. Then the following night I threw up — guess I really should have taken those anti-nausea tablets,' she says, smiling.

After her second treatment Susan realised that she was no longer functioning at her new job at *Vogue* magazine 'and more importantly I didn't want to be in the office. So I quit my job and began focusing on what mattered — living. It was such a relief to have no more office deadlines and to just concentrate on getting well and surviving — and, of course, cooking!' she adds. 'All my life, I've dived into cooking to relieve stress. I always keep a stack of cookbooks on my bedside table. Reading about a great classical dish makes me feel all is well with the world.'

Cancer, according to Susan, has given greater clarity to her world. 'How important is a messy love affair compared to a life-threatening disease? Not very!'

Then, sitting up tall on the couch and looking me straight in the eye, she tells me that somewhere along the line she had decided, 'If I am going to die, I'll die in peace. And if I am going to live, it will be a contented and useful life.'

Food, recipes, dinner parties, friends and more food are what kept Susan sane during her tough time with treatments. 'During chemo I was manic. I don't know why. I'd invite complete strangers home to dinner then spend the day cooking long and intricate dishes for them. Perhaps it gave me a focus beyond my health. Or — more bluntly — took my mind off death and instead forced me to think about living.'

After the second chemo treatment, when her hair was falling out in big tufts, it was time for a trim. 'I went over to Mona Vale and had it shorn to a fine cut all over. The hairdresser gave me two weeks before I'd be completely bald. When I looked at my shorn head, it wasn't as shocking as I thought it would be. I guess when you don't have a choice you just accept it,' she adds.

Chemotherapy is possibly the most challenging ingredient in the breast cancer treatment mix, emotionally and physically, and Susan acknowledges that there were times when it all seemed just too hard.

'I was really forced to use my mind to help me cope. I was paper thin, absolutely exhausted, had little energy and was driven mad by the hot flushes that kept me awake every night. But I would tell myself every day, over and over, that I am strong, my body is strong and my mind is strong until I believed it, despite evidence to the contrary,' she says.

After having to postpone her third dose of chemo because of a low white blood count, Susan enlisted the help of a Chinese herbalist. 'My entire life seemed consumed with looking after my body. Sometimes I wondered if I was being a mug, but desperate people do desperate things. Whenever I had to make a wish it would be, "Give me health and I will take care of the happiness."'

Although she valued the community spirit at Pittwater — a boat-access only area about 45 minutes from Sydney's CBD, where she'd settled after a long search to find a place where she might finally feel liked she belonged — Susan hadn't really told anyone about her illness. As she made her way home after the buzz cut, word soon got round. 'I hopped off the water taxi at the boatshed and one of my neighbours, Ken, glanced up from his work, nodded at my new punk look and asked me if I was going to join a rock band. I told him with no fuss, "No, just a bit of treatment."'

Susan found her peace and purpose in life alongside the sparkling blue waters of Pittwater and in a community that cared for her without intruding or overwhelming. 'Being here and finding a community that asked nothing and gave everything was, and still is, an enormous gift. This community gave me the gift of being useful and showed me how to rise above my own pond of despondency, which — in turn — allowed me to cope,' she says.

'Our community collectively got me through my darkest moments, and it is here that I discovered the happiness that I dreamed of. Assistance came from everywhere. Everyone lent a helping hand.

I'd come home with bags of groceries and someone would always come over and carry them up to the house. People dropped off the newspapers, and everyone quietly checked up on me to make sure I was okay.

'I remember one night, just before I resigned from the magazine. It was late and as I hopped onto the water taxi Annette asked me how I was. I was too tired to answer and started crying. Annette just put her arms around me and held me. Good people — that's what helps to give you strength and courage.

'I will never forget the kindness of my beautiful Buddhist friend, Adele, who stayed with me for a month after I was diagnosed. She would let me unwind, unleash my fears and uncertainties, but then gently remind me that although I was feeling bad, things could be worse. I love her dearly and will be forever grateful that she led me through the difficult times,' Susan says.

When Susan had her mastectomy, she says she didn't really mind losing her breast, but she hated the thought of having a prosthesis. 'At that time I was very skinny and so really I could have got away without wearing anything. I wore the artificial boob for months after surgery, but loathed it. I would lean over and it would fall out. Then I'd lie down and it would stay up. I gave it a name — Tom Tit. Sometimes, I'd forget to put the little pink silicon jellyfish in. It took time, but now it's just a part of the dressing routine — like pulling on a pair of socks.'

Like most women who go through cancer, Susan couldn't even conceive that life would return to normal one day. 'I had no idea how to handle life beyond chemo,' she says. 'After months of feeling like an alien, I was suddenly dumped back into mainstream living and expected to get on with life. Where do you start when you know you will have the ugly little threat of secondaries sitting on your shoulder for ever? The reality is that you never get the all-clear from cancer so the threat of a recurrence is always there.

'When I was newly diagnosed it was awful, and I didn't know if I had a month or 10 years left. That was terrifying. I remember such small things giving me hope and confidence, such as friends including me in future plans. Surely, if they believed I had a future then I must!

In time, she realised living in fear was a life half-lived. If there wasn't going to be a long time ahead, why waste it worrying about events she couldn't control? 'I found that the more useful I made myself to other people, the more I forgot about cancer.'

Not long after her operation and treatment, Susan met and eventually fell in love with the bloke next door to her home in Lovett Bay. When he asked her to marry him, she held back, though. 'I'm no prize,' she said. He replied very quickly that he thought she was. 'I have only one breast,' she told him. 'One is enough,' he said with a smile.

'For me cancer is a constant reminder that life does end, and I think because of that, I've had a far richer life in the past few years than I otherwise would have.

'I am not frightened of death now. Although I certainly was when I was first diagnosed at 49. I have looked closely at my own mortality and with my Buddhist friends' help, realised that everything that is born must die. And, truly, nothing gives you a better attitude to life than a good attitude to death.'

Susan never really asked 'Why me?' when diagnosed. 'Actually, I thought I probably brought it on myself by living a really stressful life. And I'd already been through the "Why?" phase with my husband and brother when they were diagnosed with cancer.

'I can remember seeing young kids having their chemo when I was at the hospital with my husband. They are the ones about whom you ask "Why?" So for me it was really a "What is, is,"' she says.

'Whilst I wouldn't wish this disease on anyone, sometimes the learning curve you are given, courtesy of cancer, allows you to find strength and your own brand of courage. You look for a way to cope and accept that you have to find a way to handle it, otherwise you go under. And, of course, you can't go under because every day is precious.'

Nowadays Susan's life is following a new path. The former journalist is now happily married again and comfortably ensconced in community life at Pittwater: cooking, writing and living in the moment.

'I am conscious that every day must be cherished. I try never to do anything that I don't want to do. I try not to waste a single second of my life. I've had a wobble or two but I am content in whatever space I am in — living in the moment is instinctive now.'

As I cross the waters from 'Tarrangaua' to Church Point on my way home, I am reminded of the final words from the book *Salvation Creek*:

'Susan ... discovered that not only is it never over until the last breath fades away, it quite simply gets better and better. All you have to do is ... survive!'

A MARCH MILESTONE
8 March 2004

Hello lovely FOAM ladies

I thought I'd drop you all a note to touch base and say hello.
Life for me is so busy I feel very guilty I haven't been able to
catch up with you all personally as I would like. But I hope
to see you all before I leave for Greece and the Olympics
in May. And I hear April 1st is a great day for Birthday
Champagne testing!!!!

You were all so kind last year that I am indulging in another
FOAMS UPDATE.

Today I went to my oncologist for my 3-month check-up.
Doesn't time fly? It is exactly 3 months since my last dose of
radiation and 2 months since my port-o-cath came out and I
declared myself 'officially over all cancer procedures'!

The visit to doc was quite confronting. Not because there is
anything visibly wrong with me — in fact I am a beaming ball
of energy with wild curly hair — but because she spent most of
the consultation talking about me living with my breast cancer
disease. I guess I had felt it was all done and over, but she kept
referring to my future of 'living with it' and that kind of freaked
me out. When I booked my mammogram date for next month,
I have to admit to a little, no LOTS, of nervousness.

I told her I had not thought of myself as a cancer person
any more. Should it come back, then I'll deal with it. She
then said, if it comes back as secondaries, it is fatal — not
necessarily immediately fatal, but nevertheless fatal. I hope
that 'not necessarily immediately' can mean 45 years!!!

She also gave me an interesting insight. I am struggling to lose my BIG C weight. With the combination of drugs, inactivity and early menopause, I am eager to get back to my pre-C health and fitness. Doc tells me to just accept I am a totally different person and to embrace the new person rather than trying to get back to 'where you were'. She tells me to just accept that I will never be back where I was.

I guess physically, emotionally and spiritually I am a new AnneMarie, and her words have really challenged me. But acceptance is a whole new thing — acceptance of the inevitable, or giving up????

Still, I don't want to ruin today by regretting the past and worrying about tomorrow, so day-by-day happiness for me ... and we'll see.

Yesterday I achieved the first of my post-C milestones by running (yep, RUNNING) the International Women's Day Fun. Run! I'd aimed to run non-stop and go under 35 minutes, and I ran all the way and clocked a satisfying 33.03. I have to admit it was an ugly run, especially by myself (Ness is still in Canberra), and my friends finished way ahead of me — but I did it!

I am also having my first post-C haircut this week! Those of you I haven't seen in the past few weeks, my hair is quite long (for me), dark (although I have tipped it with blonde streaks), very curly, and baby fine. I feel like a full-blown dandelion — sunny face with a wispy fly-away halo.

Thank you again to each of you for your friendship and I look forward to catching up soon.

Smile

AM

PS Ella Grace and Madeleine Kate are growing into such beautiful angels, that maybe my 'granny arms' are meant to be — for them!

ACKNOWLEDGMENTS

I would like to thank my late husband, Peter, my daughter, Vanesa, and my son, Ben, for their loving support throughout my years of treatments.

Also to Kylie and Patrick; my grandchildren, Madeleine, Ella, Matilda, Adelaide Rose and Thomas; my mother-in-law, Mette; and my sister, Jill, for always being by my side during the tough times and enjoying the great joys. And, of course, to the FOAMs, my wonderful friends, in particular Beth and Kathleen.

Thank you also to Dr Liz Kenny, who was so much more than an oncologist, and to Dr Jane Turner, whose sage advice kept me almost sane during the troubled days.

My appreciation also goes to the fabulous and professional people at HarperCollins, especially Associate Publisher Brigitta Doyle and Senior Editor Anne Reilly.